Copyright © 2024 by Dr. Su-Nui Escobar, RDN, LDN
All rights reserved.
No portion of this book may be reproduced in any form without written permission from the publisher or author except as permitted by U.S. copyright law.

Disclaimer
The information the author provides is for general informational purposes only and should not be considered a substitute for professional medical advice.

It is essential to consult with a qualified healthcare professional or physician before making any significant changes to your diet or lifestyle.

This guide is based on the expertise of a doctor in clinical nutrition and a registered dietitian. However, individual results may vary.

Credits
Images of this book are stock photos, used under proper license.

# TABLE OF CONTENTS

## 06 — Introduction
06. What does healthy eating look like when taking semaglutide?
07. What you will find in this guide

## 08 — Decoding Semaglutide
10. What is Semaglutide?
    How Semaglutide Works
    What is the Difference Between Semaglutide, Ozempic® and Wegovy®?
11. Expected Weight Loss

## 12 — Nutrition Guide for Semaglutide Users
13. The Big Picture
15. Build Your Plate
    What to Eat
23. How Much to Eat
24. Let's Talk About Protein
    The Benefits of Protein for Weight Loss
25. Calculating Your Protein Needs
26. How to Reach Your Protein Goals
27. Protein Shakes, Powder and Bars
28. A Note for Vegetarians
    Fiber
29. Fluids
30. Alcohol
32. Create a Calorie Deficit to Lose Weight
    Calculate Your Calorie Needs
34. Tracking Calories
35. Supplements
    Vitamins and Minerals
36. Probiotics
38. Eating Out
39. Tips for Eating Out

## 40 — Semaglutide Side Effects (And How to Get Relief)

40. Side Effects
42. How Long Side Effects Last
43. Constipation
    Essential Tips for Easing Constipation
44. Foods That Relieve Constipation
    Additional Nutrition and Lifestyle Tips to Improve Constipation
45. Over-the-Counter Remedies
46. When to Talk to Your Doctor
47. Diarrhea
    Changes in Your Diet
48. Over-the-Counter Medications
    When to Call Your Doctor
49. Nausea
    Changes in Your Diet
50. Natural Remedies to Relieve Nausea
    Foods Easier to Tolerate
51. Other Helpful Tips
    When to Call Your Doctor
52. Burping
    Changes in Diet
53. When to See a Doctor
54. Fatigue

## 55 — Other Common Concerns

56. Not Eating Enough
57. Tips to Eat Enough
58. Not Losing Weight
59. Possible Reasons Why you are not Losing Weight

## 60 — Move More

How Much Exercise Do You Need?
61. Cardiovascular Exercises
62. Strength Training
    Flexibility
63. Tips to Incorporate Physical Activity

## 64 — Mindful Eating

What is Mindful Eating?
65. Benefits of Mindful Eating
Mindful Eating Checklist

## 67 — What Happens When You Stop Taking Semaglutide?

68. Tips to Keep the Weight Off

## 70 — Meal Ideas

72. Breakfast
73. Lunch
74. Dinner
75. Snack
76. Recipes breakfast
83. Recipes Lunch
91. Recipes Dinner

# Easy-to-Follow Nutrition Guide to Lose Weight on Semaglutide

Semaglutide—also known by the brand names Ozempic® and Wegovy®—has become immensely popular in recent years due to its effectiveness in promoting weight loss.

The amount of weight people can lose on semaglutide is remarkable!

However, it's important to note that it's not a magical solution; diet and exercise remain key in optimizing weight loss, maintaining your muscle mass, and minimizing side effects.

**What does healthy eating look like when taking semaglutide?**

As a doctor in clinical nutrition and registered dietitian I quickly realized that losing weight with the aid of semaglutide is a whole new game. Semaglutide users don't require complex diets. Instead, they benefit from simple eating patterns that prioritize the right foods to achieve their goals, maintain muscle mass, minimize side effects, and feel fantastic.

The needs of a person taking semaglutide for weight loss are very different from those seeking to lose weight without the aid of obesity medication.

Also, soon after you start taking the medication, it's important to start establishing sustainable healthy eating and exercise habits. Obesity medications are designed for long-term use; however, their effectiveness may decrease over time, and many factors may lead you to discontinue the medication. Without solid habits in place, weight regain is almost certain.

I took all of this into consideration when writing this guide, and I also seek to provide you with options to tailor the advice to your lifestyle.

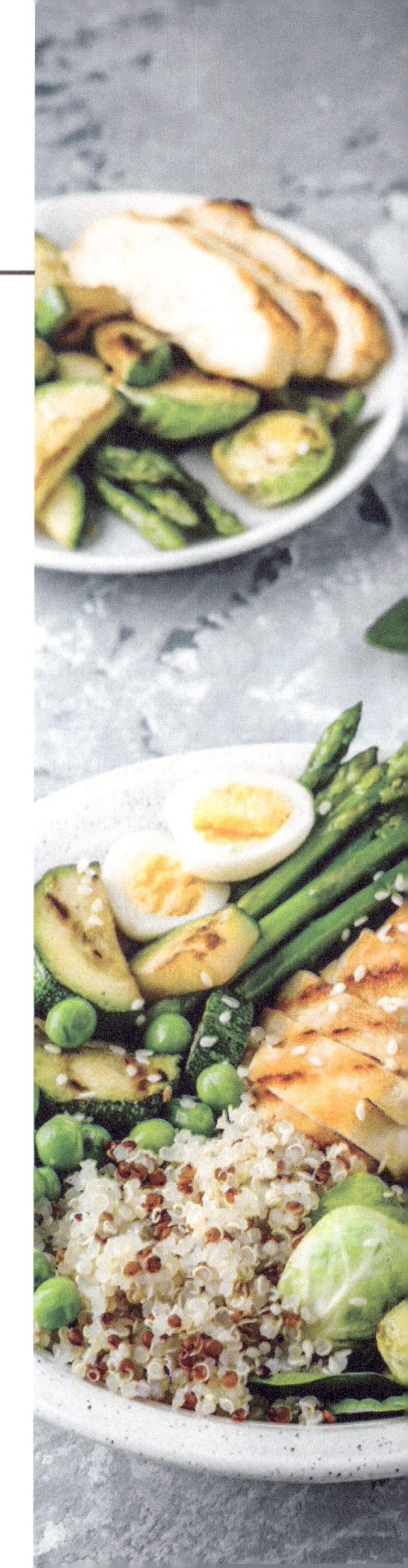

Copyright © 2024 by Dr. Su-Nui Escobar, RDN, LDN

## What you will find in this guide:

- An easy-to-follow plan to help you build your meals with the right foods.
- A comprehensive list of foods broken down into foods you can eat more often, foods to limit, and foods to eat rarely or avoid altogether.
- Nutrition and lifestyle tips to help you minimize side effects
- A guide to physical activity
- A mindful eating check list

But before we begin, let's look at what semaglutide is and how it works, which will help you understand the eating style you need.

# Decoding
# Semaglutide

# What is Semaglutide?

Semaglutide is a medication used in the treatment of type 2 diabetes and obesity.

The FDA recommends the use of the medication along with healthy eating and exercise.

## What is the difference between semaglutide, Ozempic®, and Wegovy®?

Semaglutide is the active ingredient in Ozempic® and Wegovy® which are the brand names of the semaglutide manufactured by Novo Nordisk. The first one is approved for diabetes, while the second is specifically approved for weight loss.

Currently, in 2024, the no generic version of semaglutide and the medication is difficult to find. When this happens with any medication, the FDA approves compound pharmacies to make versions of the drug. However, these versions of semaglutide do not have the same testing and are not FDA-approved.

# How Semaglutide Works

This weight-loss drug works by imitating the actions of a hormone called GLP-1, produced by your gut and your brain.

This hormone acts in response to eating to decrease the appetite. It also slows down the rate at which the stomach empties, making you feel fuller for longer and reducing hunger. It helps to decrease insulin resistance, enabling the body to use stored fat for energy more efficiently. This also results in fewer cravings and better use of food for energy instead of fat.

Lastly, the action of GLP-1 on your brain can also help you regulate your appetite.

By combining these effects, semaglutide helps people eat less and feel less hungry, ultimately leading to weight loss.

## Expected Weight Loss

It's important to have realistic expectations when it comes to weight loss to avoid unnecessary frustration. In clinical trials, semaglutide has helped people lose an average of 15-17% of their initial body weight.

Some people lose more, some lose less. There are many factors involved including initial weight, diet, exercise, age, gender, and many others.

Moreover, some people respond very quickly to the medication and start losing weight at the lowest dose. Others don't start losing weight until they reach the highest dose.

Also keep in mind that experts consider a weight loss of between ½ to 2 pounds a week healthy and sustainable.

# Nutrition Guide for Semaglutide Users

The main nutrition goals for semaglutide users include:

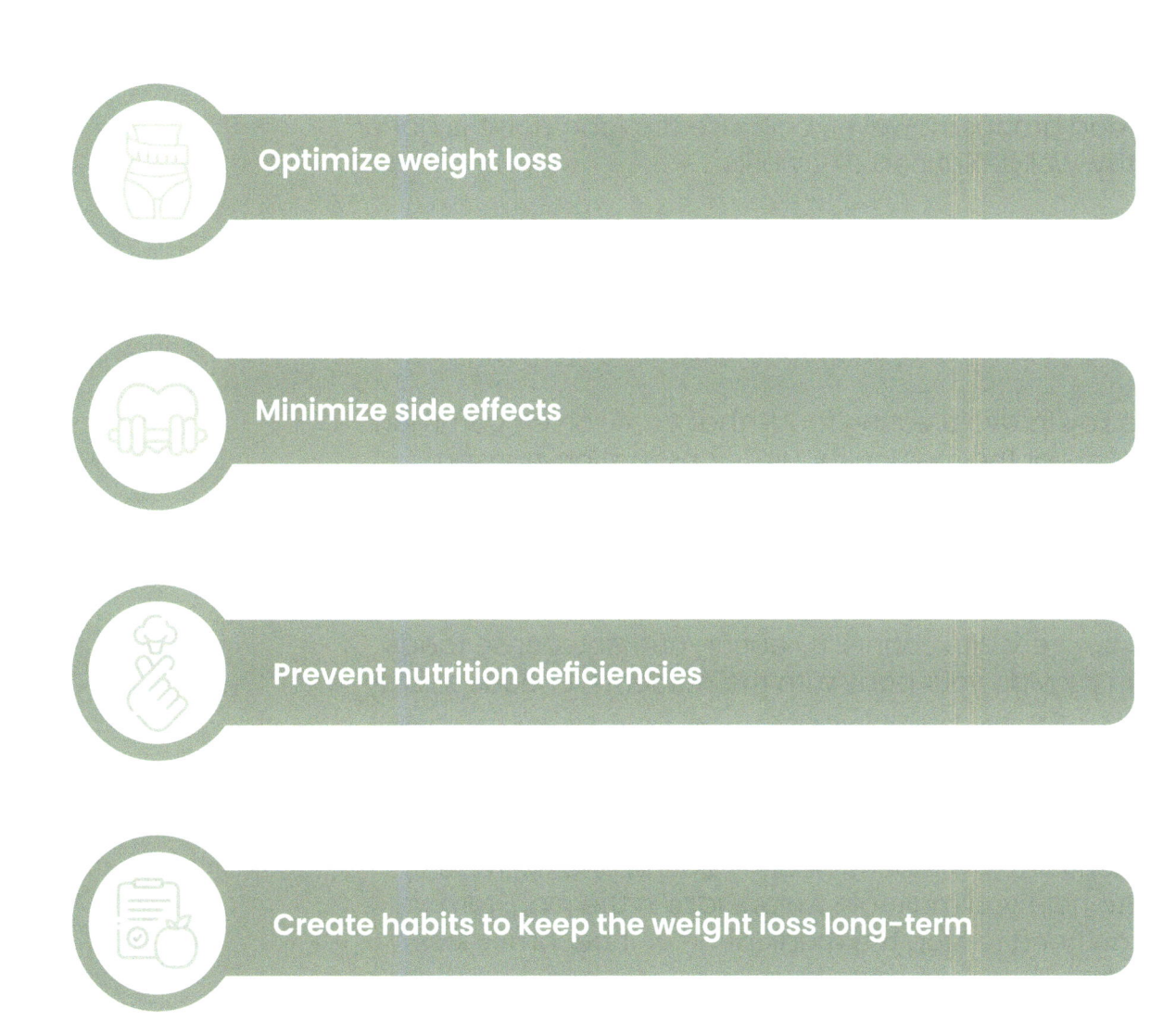

- Optimize weight loss
- Minimize side effects
- Prevent nutrition deficiencies
- Create habits to keep the weight loss long-term

# The Big Picture

For weight loss and health, it's essential to eat a well-balanced diet. This means eating a variety of foods in the right proportion to get the essential nutrients your body needs. This can be difficult for people used to restricting entire food groups. However, because the food noise is gone, a healthy, well-balanced diet works!

Eating healthy also means avoiding processed and refined foods, limiting unhealthy fats and sugars, and increasing your consumption of fruit, vegetables, whole grains, lean meats, and dairy products (optional).

It's also key to avoid eating foods that can worsen common side effects of the medication, like constipation, nausea, diarrhea, and other GI symptoms.

Moreover, semaglutide can make people lose their appetite to the point that eating becomes difficult. When this happens, every bite counts. By eating nutrient-dense foods, you can provide your body with the nutrients it needs to stay healthy.

It's important to remember that many people regain weight once they stop this medication. For that reason, it's important to concentrate on creating healthy eating and exercise habits to help you maintain weight loss in the long-term in case you need to stop the medication or it becomes less effective.

In addition to these considerations, it's also important to drink plenty of water to stay hydrated.

This guide is easy to follow because easy works. Now that you're taking semaglutide, you can forget about elaborate diets; the focus is on the quality of your meals. Semaglutide will help reduce the food noise that made you fail in the past.

This nutrition guide is divided into three main sections. In the first section, you'll find an easy-to-follow method for building a healthy plate. The second part offers lists of foods to enjoy frequently, those to enjoy in moderation, and those to limit. The third section outlines appropriate portion sizes.

You will also find information on protein, calories, and supplements.

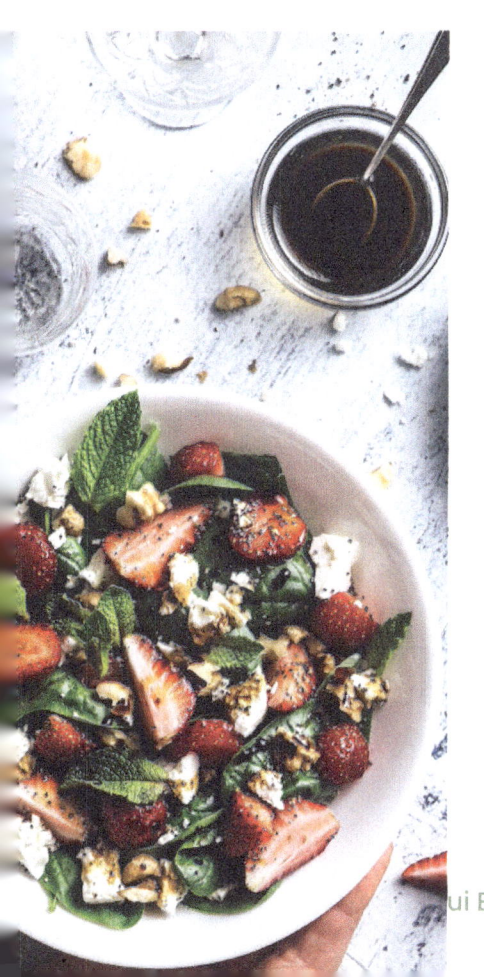

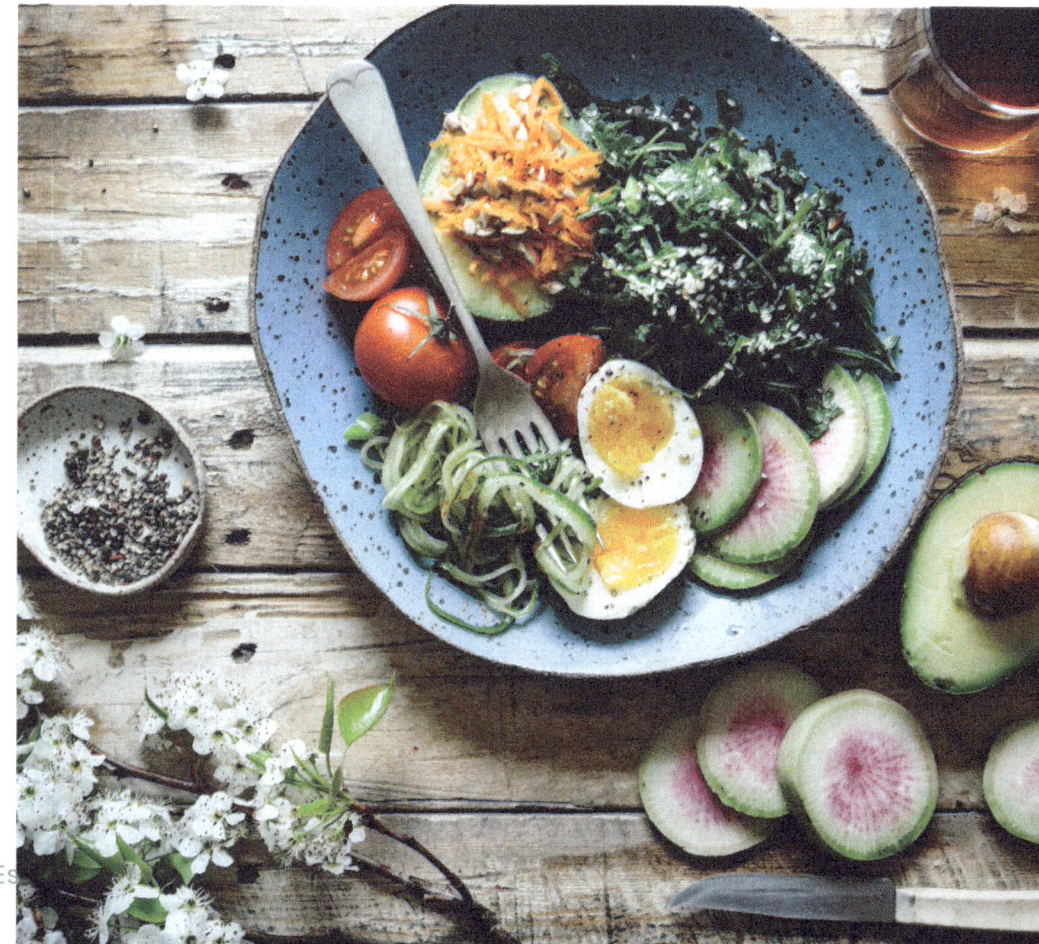

# Build Your **Plate**

### Start with protein

Make protein the center of your meal. Aim for 25-30 grams of protein per meal (3-4 ounces).

Select most of your protein from the green section of the food list you will find in the next section.

Building your plate around protein can help you lose weight while maintaining your muscle mass and will provide you with essential nutrients.

The portion sizes in this guide will make it easy to consume the protein you need. But if you want to personalize your food intake to your specific needs, refer to page 25, where I guide you step by step in how to calculate your requirements. Those with higher protein needs can add a high-protein snack or increase protein intake during meals.

> **Note for people living outside the United States (using the metric system).**
>
> If you're used to weighing food in grams, you might find this recommendation confusing. However, it's important to note that grams of protein are not the same as grams of weight.
> For instance, one large egg contains only 6 grams of protein, while approximately 120 grams of salmon provide about 25 grams of protein. Therefore, eating around 120-150 grams of chicken, fish, or beef will supply you with the protein you need per meal.

### Add vegetables

Vegetables are a wonderful way to add nutrients, flavor, and volume to your meals. Most important, vegetables are high in fiber, which can help minimize common side effects of weight loss medication

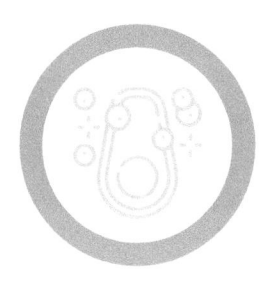

### Include healthy fats

Adding healthy fats to your meals can help you feel satiated and full after eating. You can use the fat to cook, as part of salad dressings, or to add flavor to your meal.

In this guide, you can count cheese and salad dressings as fat.

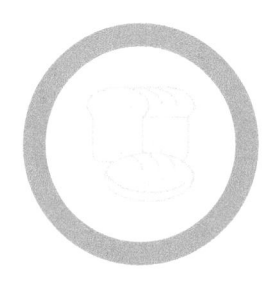

### Incorporate a moderate amount of healthy carbs.

A healthy carbohydrate is one that is high in fiber and that provides good nutrition.

In this guide, we suggest eating carbs for breakfast and lunch to make meals easier. Keep dinners low-carb to help control your carbohydrate intak overall.

So, your meals will look like this:

| | |
|---|---|
| Breakfast | 1 protein + vegetables or fruit + 1 fat + 1 carbohydrate |
| Lunch | 1 protein + vegetables + 1 fat + 1 carbohydrate |
| Dinner | 1 protein + vegetables + 1 fat + 1 carbohydrate (optional) |
| Snack (optional) | 1 protein or fat + 1 vegetable, protein, or carbohydrate |

The next section will provide an extensive list of the best foods to choose for weight loss and the ones you want to limit.

You will find **meal ideas** at the end of this guide.

# How to Use **This List**

---

This list is divided into the following food categories:

- Protein
- Vegetables and fruit
- Fat
- Carbohydrates

Each category is then divided into three colors: red, yellow, and green.

Green means **go**. Eat from the green list most of the time. Choose foods from the green section for all your meals.

Yellow means **caution**. Eat foods in the yellow list occasionally, ideally only 3 to 5 times a week.

Red means **stop**. Completely avoid or limit foods in the red column.

# Food List

| Go - Eat every day if desired | Caution - Eat 2-3 meals per week | Red - Limit to twice a month |
|---|---|---|

## PROTEINS

| Go | Caution | Red |
|---|---|---|
| Buffalo | Beef, lean | Bacon |
| Burger, vegetarian | Chicken, thighs and legs | Chicken, fried |
| Chicken breast | Pork | Chorizo |
| Clams | Sardines, canned in oil | Fish, fried |
| Crab | Tuna, canned in oil | Hot dog |
| Eggs | Turkey | Milanese |
| Fish | Turkey bacon | Sausage |
| Lobster | Turkey sausage | Ribs |
| Octopus | Veal | Yogurt with > 5 g of added sugar |
| Pork, lean | Greek yogurt made with whole milk | - |
| Salmon | - | - |
| Sardines, in water | - | - |
| Scallops | - | - |
| Shrimp | - | - |
| Tempeh | - | - |
| Turkey, lean | - | - |
| Tofu | - | - |

## NON-STARCHY VEGETABLES

| Go | Caution | Red |
|---|---|---|
| Artichoke and artichoke hearts | Artichoke and artichoke hearts, canned | Vegetables in cheese sauce |
| Asparagus | Canned vegetables | Vegetables tempura |
| Beets | Fermented vegetables | Fried vegetables |
| Bok choy | Heart of palm packed in water | - |
| Broccoli | Kimchi | - |

Copyright © 2024 by Dr. Su-Nui Escobar, RDN, LDN

| | | |
|---|---|---|
| Brussel sprouts | Pickled beets | - |
| Cabbage | Sauerkraut | - |
| Carrots | Sun Dried tomatoes with olive oil | - |
| Cauliflower | - | - |
| Cauliflower rice | - | - |
| Celery | - | - |
| Collard greens | - | - |
| Cucumber | - | - |
| Jicama | - | - |
| Kale | - | - |
| Mushrooms, all kinds, fresh | - | - |
| Okra | - | - |
| Onions and shallots | - | - |
| Peppers (bell, chille, and other kinds) | - | - |
| Radishes | - | - |
| Leafy greens | - | - |
| Spinach | - | - |
| Squash | - | - |
| Swiss chard | - | - |
| Tomatoes | - | - |
| Zucchini | - | - |

## FATS

**FATS AND OILS**

| | | |
|---|---|---|
| Almond butter | Butter | Bacon |
| Avocado | Safflower oil | Coconut milk, canned |
| Avocado oil | Salad dressing, creamy | Half-and-half cream |
| Canola oil | Soybean oil | Lard |
| Flaxseed oil | Sour cream, light | Shortening, solid |

| | | |
|---|---|---|
| Olives | - | Sour cream, regular |
| Olive oil | - | - |
| Peanut butter | - | - |
| Peanut oil | - | - |
| Sesame oil | - | - |
| Vinaigrettes | - | - |

## NUTS AND SEEDS

| | | |
|---|---|---|
| Almonds | Any roasted or salted nuts and seeds | Nuts roasted with sugar |
| Almond butter | - | - |
| Brazil nuts | - | - |
| Cashews | - | - |
| Chia seeds | - | - |
| Flaxseeds | - | - |
| Peanuts | - | - |
| Peanut butter, no sugar added | - | - |
| Pecans | - | - |
| Pistachios | - | - |
| Pumpkin seeds | - | - |
| Sesame seeds | - | - |
| Sunflower seeds | - | - |
| Walnuts | - | - |

## CHEESE

| | | |
|---|---|---|
| Cheese, thin slice | Cheese, ricotta | Cheese, proccesed |
| Cheese, ricotta, part skim | Cheese | Cream cheese, regular |
| - | Cream cheese, low-fat | - |

# CARBOHYDRATES
## BREAD, TORTILLAS, WRAPS

| | | |
|---|---|---|
| Bagel-thin whole wheat | Bagel | Bakery products |
| Baguette, whole wheat | Baguette | Cakes |
| Bread, whole wheat | Biscuit | Cinnamon roll |
| Corn tortilla | Bread, white | Croissants |
| Oatmeal bread | Hamburger bun | Cupcakes |
| Pancake, whole wheat or oatmeal | Pancake | Danish |
| Pita, whole wheat | Pita, white | Donuts |
| Sprouted bread | - | Focaccia |
| Whole wheat tortilla | - | Garlic bread |
| Wrap-low carb | - | Hawaiian rolls |
| Zero carbs tortillas | - | Muffins |

## CEREALS, GRAINS, PASTA, AND RICE

| | | |
|---|---|---|
| Barley | Brown rice pasta | Cereal ready-to-eat with sugar |
| Black bean pasta | Cereals with less than 8 grams of sugar | Fried rice |
| Bran cereal | Granola, low-fat | Lasagna |
| Brown rice | Granola bars | Pasta salad |
| Buckwheat | Gnocchi | Pasta with creamy sauces |
| Chickpea pasta | Egg noodles | - |
| Farro | Flavored oatmeal, ready-to-eat | - |
| Lentil pasta | White rice | - |
| Oats | Pasta with tomato sauce | - |
| Pasta whole-wheat | - | - |
| Quinoa | - | - |

Copyright © 2024 by Dr. Su-Nui Escobar, RDN, LDN

| | | |
|---|---|---|
| Shirataki noodles | - | - |
| Tabbouleh | - | - |
| Zucchini noodles | - | - |
| Spaghetti squash | - | - |

## BEANS, PEAS, LENTILS, AND OTHER LEGUMES

| | | |
|---|---|---|
| Beans-all types | Refried beans, fat-free | Baked beans, |
| Garbanzo | - | Pork & beans |
| Lentils | - | Refried beans |
| Split peas | - | - |
| Peas | - | - |

## FRUITS

| | | |
|---|---|---|
| Fresh fruit | Dried fruit, no sugar | Dried fruit with sugar |
| Unsweetened frozen fruit | - | Fruit juice |
| - | - | Fruit, canned |

## CONDIMENTS AND SAUCES

| | | |
|---|---|---|
| Apple cider vinegar | Agave | Alfredo sauce |
| Balsamic vinegar | Chimichurri | BBQ sauce |
| Coconut Amino | Curry sauce | Creamy salad dressings |
| Dijon mustard | Pesto | Mayonnaise |
| Fresh salsa | Sugar-free syrup | Pancake syrup |
| Hot sauce | Plum sauce | Sweet and sour sauce |
| Miso | Light salad dressings | Vodka sauce |
| Mustard | Teriyaki sauce | - |
| Soy sauce (low sodium) | - | - |
| Vinegar | - | - |

Copyright © 2024 by Dr. Su-Nui Escobar, RDN, LDN

# How Much to Eat

You are less likely to overeat while on semaglutide, so keeping your portions under control is the easy part. However, being aware of your portion sizes can improve your success. There are two ways in which you can measure the quantity of food you consume. The most accurate form of measurement is the weight of the food. But a quick and easy measurement is your hand.

**Protein:**
- 3 to 6 ounces per meal
- 3 to 6 ounces = the palm of your hand

**Non-starchy vegetables:** unlimited

**Carbohydrates:**
- 1 cup or 30-45 grams
- 1 cup = the fist of your hand
- Bread, tortillas, wraps = 1 large or 2 small

**Fat** = 1 tablespoon
- For avocados, you can have 2 tablespoons
- 1 tablespoon = the tip of your thumb

**Tip:** If you are not very hungry but you know you need to eat, start by eating your protein and vegetables or fruit and leave the carbohydrates to end.

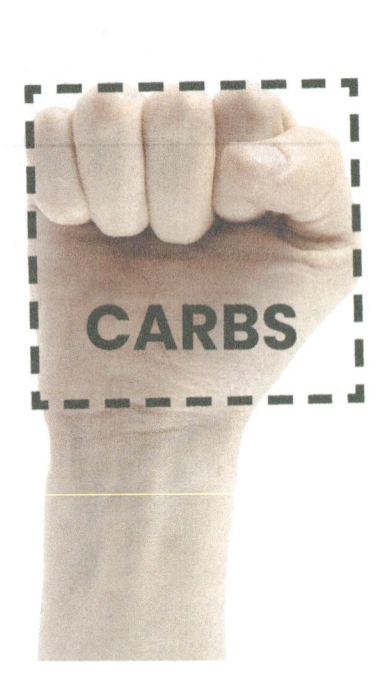

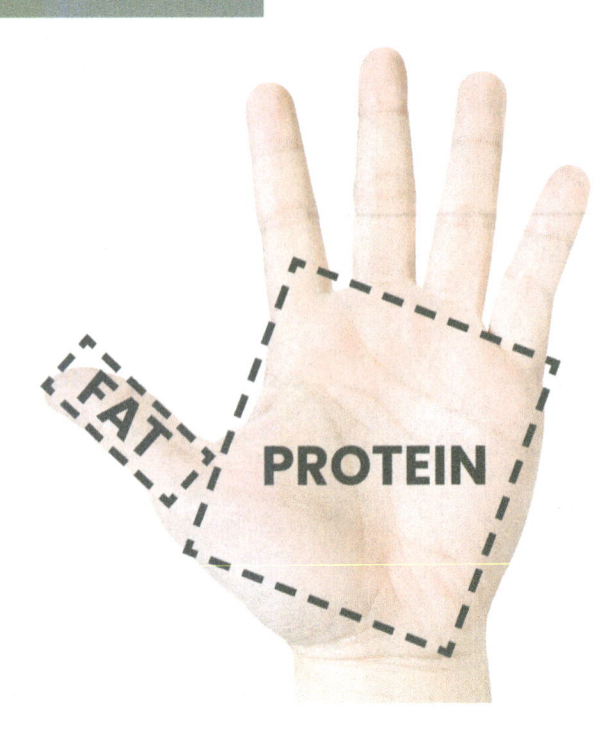

CARBS

FAT  PROTEIN

# Let's Talk About **Protein**

**The Benefits of Protein for Weight Loss**
Protein is, without a doubt, a micronutrient you need to pay special attention to because of its many benefits for weight loss, including:

- **Preserves muscle mass:**
  When you lose weight, you lose fat and muscle. Eating an adequate amount of protein (and exercising) helps maintain muscle tissue. This can help you to look toned and healthy. This is important at any age but essential if you are older than 40.

- **Burns more calories:**
  Protein has a higher thermic effect compared to fats and carbohydrates. This means your body burns more calories processing protein-rich foods, contributing to overall calorie expenditure. A body with more lean muscle also increases your basal metabolic rate (the number of calories you burn at rest).

- **Supports muscle growth and repair:**
  Regular exercise combined with an adequate protein intake can help you build and maintain lean muscle mass. But don't worry—you will not look like a body builder unless you train specifically for that!

- **Supports the effect of semaglutide:**
  Protein can also make you feel fuller for longer, reducing the likelihood of overeating or snacking in between meals. It also helps control the appetite and satiety hormones.

- **Helps with weight maintenance:**
  After reaching your goal weight, eating enough protein can help maintain your new weight by keeping you feeling full and satisfied while providing essential nutrients for overall health.

It's important to note that while protein is essential for weight loss, it's also important to maintain a well-balanced diet that includes a variety of nutrients from fruits, whole grains, and healthy fats.

Additionally, individual protein needs vary based on many factors.

# Calculating Your **Protein Needs**

Let's calculate your protein needs.

While eating according to this guide will get you close to your goal, knowing your protein needs can help you tailor the plan to your specific needs.

Please remember that more information is necessary to provide you with an exact number but this calculation can give you a good idea of your personalized needs.

**Step 1:**
Calculate your weight in kilograms: simply divide your weight in pounds by 2.2.

Example:
220 pounds divided by 2.2 = 100kg

**Step 2:**
Multiply your weight in kilograms by 1.34. This will give you an estimate of your protein needs for the day.

Example:
100kg x 1.34 = 134 grams

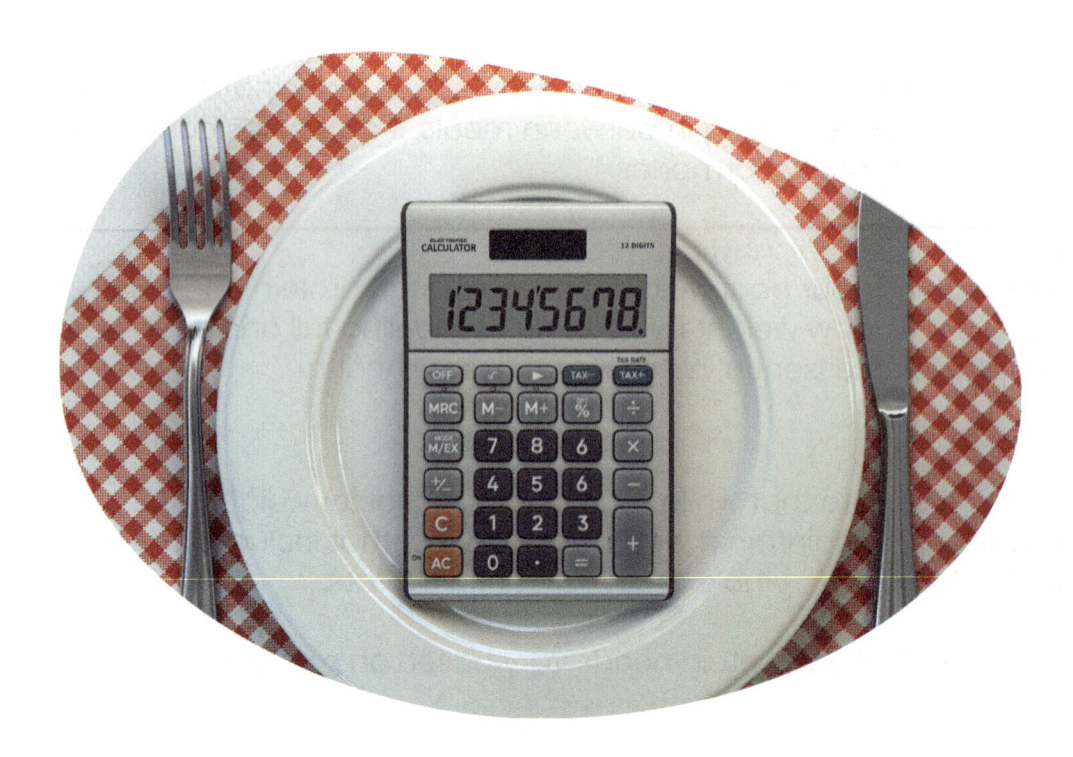

# How to reach your **Protein Goals**

In this book, we encourage you to aim for 25 to 30 grams of protein per meal. If you eat three meals, you will consume 75 to 90 grams of protein a day, along with additional protein found in items we don't typically consider primary protein sources, like carbohydrates and some vegetables.

So, by simply incorporating protein sources into all your meals, you'll likely meet or come close to your protein intake goal.

However, if you have higher protein needs, ensure your snacks also contain protein or increase the protein content of your meals. Getting enough protein is honestly not difficult; it's just a matter of being mindful of your food choices.

Find a list of foods high in protein that you enjoy from the food list previously mentioned in this guide.

> **A note for vegetarians**
>
> Eating enough plant-based protein can be more challenging, so it's very important to be mindful of your protein intake in every meal. Also, choose carbohydrates that can add protein to your diet such as quinoa, beans, garbanzo and other legumes.

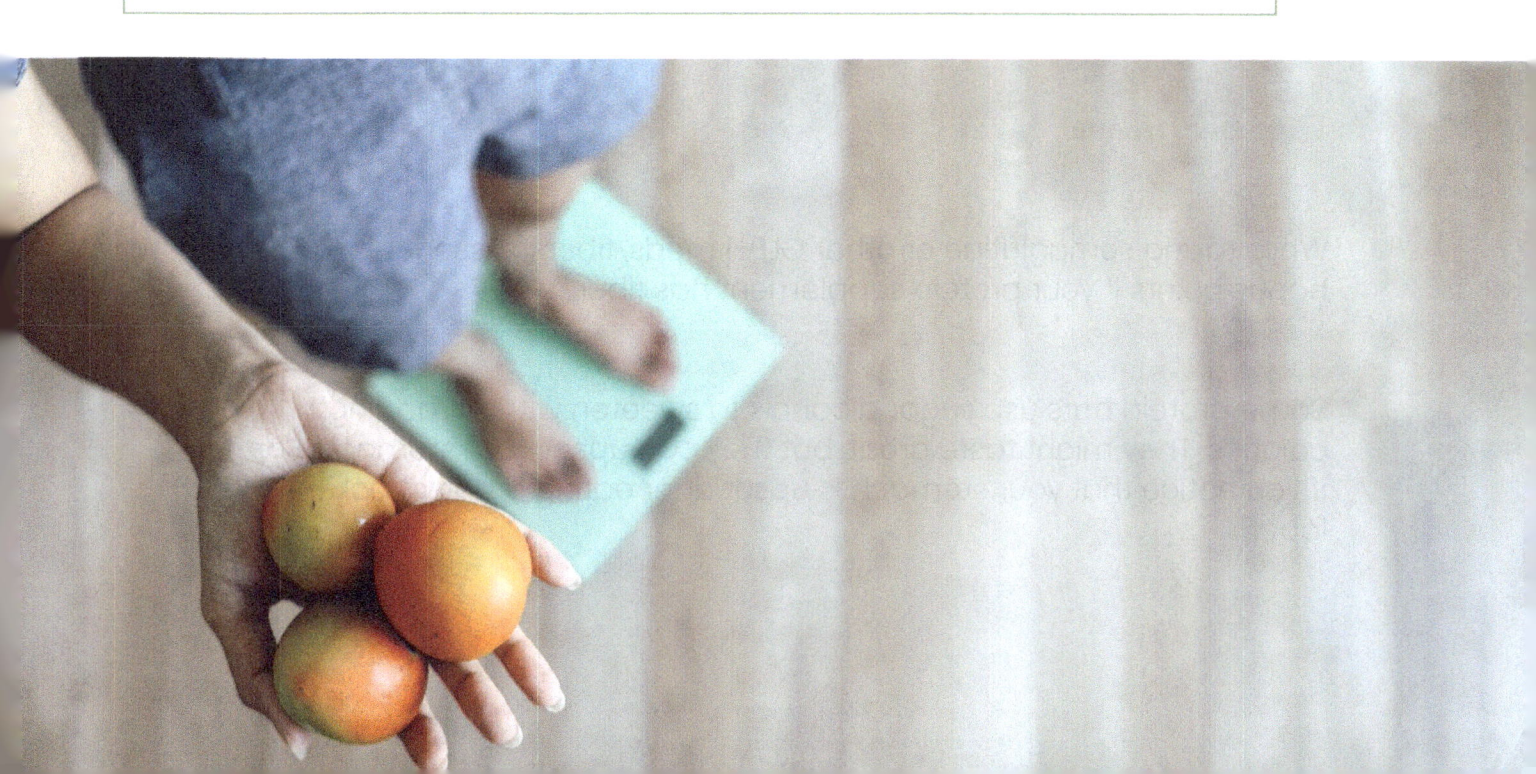

# Protein Shakes, Powder and Bars

Protein shakes and bars are a great option for GLP-1 users. While I encourage getting protein from real foods, people taking semaglutide might face challenges like reduced hunger, nausea, or a busy lifestyle. So, having a protein bar or shake can help meet your protein and energy needs quickly and easily.

## How to Select Protein Supplement

**The non-negotiables**

- **Check protein content:**
  Look for options with at least 10 to 20 grams of protein per serving to ensure you are getting enough.

- **Watch calories:**
  Because your goal is weight loss, keep an eye on calories, and select those with **less than 250 calories** per serving. However, if your protein shake, bar, or powder is part of a meal or snack, you might want to choose one with fewer calories.

- **Keep an eye on sugar:**
  Avoid those with excessive added sugar, which can hinder your weight loss efforts.

**You can also review**

- **Fiber content:**
  While taking semaglutide or other GLP-1 meds, fiber is essential! So, bonus points if your protein supplement has fiber.

- **Sugar alcohols:**
  Some protein bars use sugar alcohols to sweeten without adding calories. They might taste great, but they can upset your stomach. So, if you notice that your stomach is upset after eating a bar, check the label.

# Fiber

Fiber is another crucial nutrient for semaglutide users—for one thing, it aids digestion, but it also minimizes side effects. Additionally, fiber helps with weight loss by keeping you satisfied for longer.

How much **fiber** do you need?

The Academy of Nutrition and Dietetics recommends that women aim for 25 grams of fiber per day and men, 38 grams.

Foods that are high in fiber.

| | |
|---|---|
| Legumes | Beans, lentils, chickpeas, split peas, and other legumes. |
| Vegetables | All vegetables, but make sure to include raw vegetables as they contain a higher amount of fiber than cooked ones or those made into juices. |
| Fruits | All fruits. Include foods that have skin on, like apples. |
| Whole Grains | Whole what bread (read labels to find one high in fiber), quinoa, brown rice, oats, and others. |
| Nuts and Seeds | Flaxseeds, chia seeds, almonds, cashews, pistachios, and others. |

As you will notice, these foods are included in your nutrition guide.

# Fluids

Drinking enough fluids is essential for overall health, playing a key role in numerous bodily functions. When it comes to semaglutide users, drinking water and other fluids can support digestion and help prevent or minimize some of the medication's side effects.

How much **water** do you need to drink?

The National Academy of Medicine recommends 13 cups of daily fluids for healthy men and 9 cups for women, with a cup being 8 ounces (250 ml). However, several factors can increase your fluid requirements. For instance, if you're physically active or live in warmer climates, you may need more.

Staying hydrated is key for keeping your bathroom visit smooth sailing! But water is not your only hydration hero.

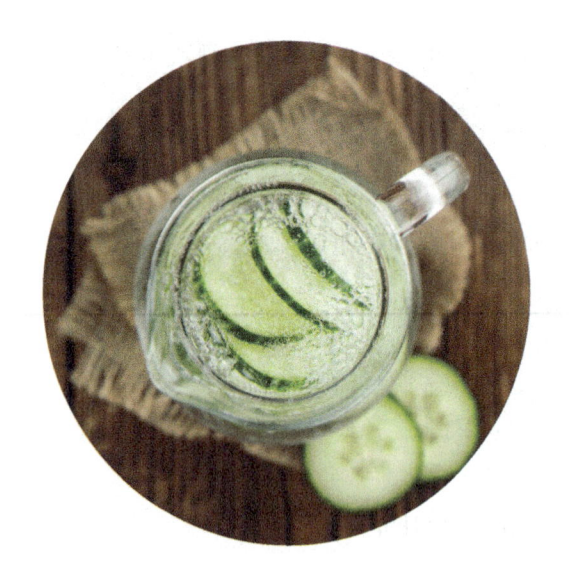

### What else counts as fluids?

Herbal teas, milk, sparkling water, soups, and smoothies can also provide those valuable fluids. Just keep an eye out for added sugars and stick to low-calorie choices.

Of course, water should still be your primary go-to drink. To make your water more appealing, try tossing in some fruits or veggies for a tasty twist! Imagine you are in a fancy spa drinking water with slices of cucumber and lime.

# Alcohol

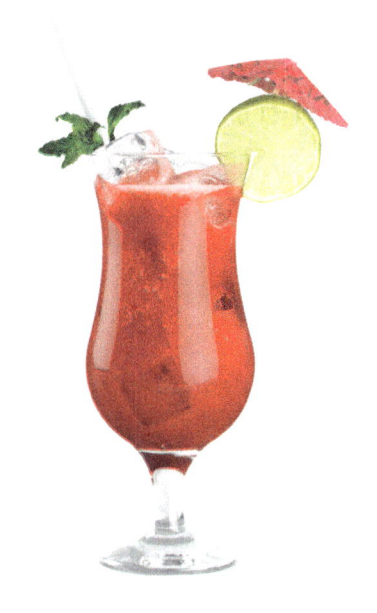

Alcohol can have a significant **negative impact** on your weight-loss efforts. However, you might notice that the desire for alcohol decreases while on semaglutide. In fact, researchers are now investigating how or why semaglutide decreases the desire for alcoholic beverages and whether this happens to most people.

Because we don't know yet where we stand with alcohol and semaglutide, let's review how alcohol can impact weight loss and—most important—the alcoholic and non-alcoholic alternatives to high-calorie alcoholic drinks.

**How alcohol impacts your weight loss:**

- Alcoholic beverages **can add calories**, making weight loss more challenging.

- Drinking **can lower inhibitions**, leading to poor food choices or overeating under its influence.

- Alcohol **can disrupt sleep**, which is an important part of weight loss. Affects digestion.

For GLP-1 users, alcohol can also worsen some side effects, such as nausea.

It's wise to limit or avoid alcohol during your weight-loss journey; and if you choose to drink, remember that **moderation is the key**. Moderation is defined as one drink a day for women and two for men.

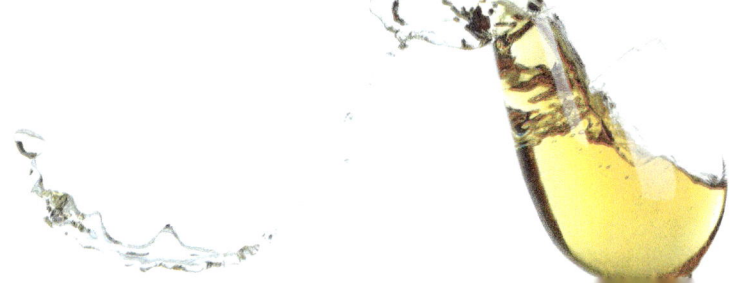

# Low-Calorie Alcohol Beverages

Fortunately, there are many low-calorie alternatives to high-calorie alcoholic beverages, including:

- Vodka soda
- Light beer
- Gin and diet tonic
- Rum and Diet Coke
- Champagne or sparkling wine
- Alcoholic drinks using soda as a mixer
- Skinny cocktails
- White wine spritzer

# Non-Alcoholic Alternatives

If you enjoy the ambiance of a bar or restaurant but prefer non-alcoholic options, navigating the drinks menu can sometimes be challenging. Here are a few ideas for non-alcoholic beverages that still deliver the experience of a cocktail, making it easier for you to enjoy your time out.

- Ask for the mocktail menu
- Virgin mojito
- Muddled fruit and club soda
- Sparkling water with cranberry juice
- Cranberry spritz
- Sparkling water with lemon or lime
- Non-alcoholic wine
- Non-alcoholic beer

You can also try these alternatives at home.

# Healthy Alternatives to Alcohol:

- Kombucha
- Apple cider vinegar drink
- Flavored sprakling water

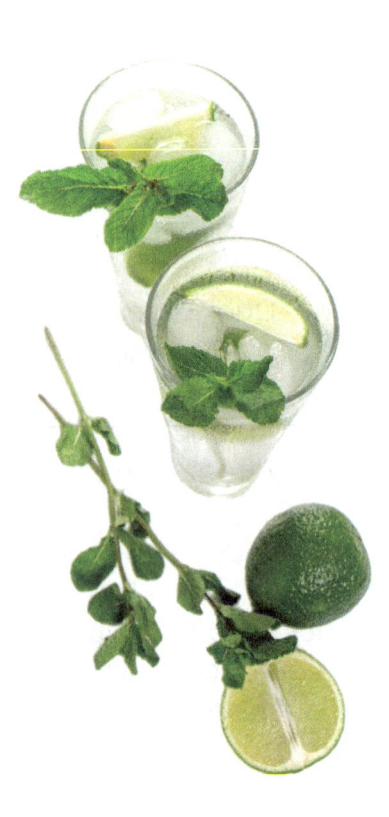

# **Create** a Calorie Deficit to Lose Weight

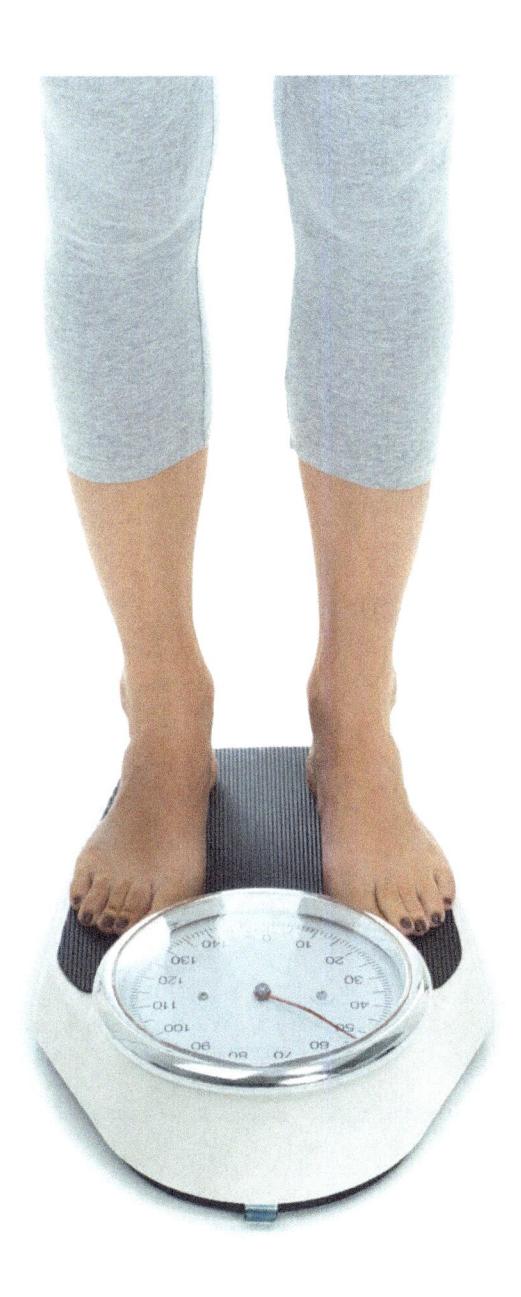

You generally don't need to focus on calories while on semaglutide in order to successfully lose weight. However, for some people, knowing their daily calorie needs makes it easier to create the deficit they need to lose weight. It can also be good to have this information if you're not losing weight to ensure you're not overeating.

## Calculate Your Calorie Needs

To lose weight, you need to eat fewer calories than you use (create a calorie deficit). The number of calories you require is based on your age, gender, weight, height, and level of physical activity.

**One very accurate method dietitians use to calculate dietary needs is by utilizing equations such as the Mifflin St Jeor.** You can easily find a Mifflin St Jeor calculator online.

## STEP 1

Find a Mifflin St Jeor calculator online and add your gender, age, weight, height. Then, the formula will also ask your activity level.

If using pounds and inches to calculate the equation, make sure that the online calculator is set for the imperial system; and if using kilograms and centimeters, ensure it's set to the metric system. Also, If you're not sure about what gender to use, add the gender you were assigned at birth.

## STEP 2

Subtract 250-500 from the total to promote weight loss. This is the number of calories you need to eat each day to lose weight.

As you lose weight, you will need to calculate your needs again. I suggest you do this every 3 months.

---

If you're good at math, maybe you'd prefer to calculate your needs manually. Here is the formula:

- **Men:** 10 x weight in kg + 6.25 x height in cm - 5 x age in years + 5
- **Women:** 10 x weight in kg + 6.25 x height in cm - 5 x age in years -161

If you use pounds, you can calculate your weight in kilograms by dividing your weight in pounds by 2.2. To calculate your height in centimeters, multiply your height in inches by 2.54.

Now that you have **this** number, you multiply it by your physical activity level:

| Activity Level | | |
|---|---|---|
| Sedentary | Little to no exercise | 1.2 |
| Lightly active | Lite exercise/sport 1-3 days a week | 1.375 |
| Moderately active | Moderate exercise/sports 3-5 days a week | 1.55 |
| Very active | Intense exercise/sports 6-7 days per week | 1.75 |
| Extra active | Very intense exercise/sports and physical job | 1.9 |

Then subtract **250-500** from the total per day to promote weight loss.

## Tracking Calories

Tracking calories can help you stay in a calorie deficit, give you an insight into your eating habits and give you freedom to choose new foods. However, it's not for everyone and can be time consuming. It is really your choice; I see it working very well for some people, but **it's not a must.**

### Can you use an app to track calories?

Yes, you can use apps like MyFitnessPal, Lose It, or Chronometer to simplify calorie tracking. They will determine your calorie requirements and enable you to monitor the calories you consume.

However, tracking calories is not necessary. While on weight-loss medication, you will be far less likely to overeat. But if you're not losing weight, looking at the calories you're consuming can help you understand what prevents you from losing weight.

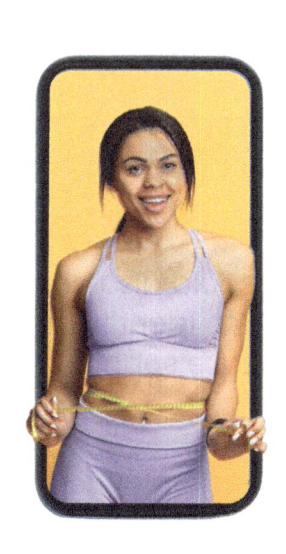

# Supplements

Getting most of your nutrients from food is the best way to nourish your body. However, people taking semaglutide for weight loss have a few challenges, so it might be useful to consider supplements.

## Vitamins and minerals

To begin, obese individuals often have nutrient deficiencies including:

- Iron
- Zinc
- Calcium
- Magnesium
- Copper
- Folate
- Potassium
- Selenium
- Vitamins A
- Vitamin B12

Additionally, individuals taking semaglutide might not eat enough or have a sufficiently varied diet, leading to inadequate intake of vitamins and minerals. While the initial step is to improve eating habits by consuming enough nutritious food and focusing on quality, taking vitamin and mineral supplements may be necessary.

For most people, taking a multivitamin is a good idea. However, it's always best to discuss with your prescribing physician whether it's suitable for you.

You could also consider getting a nutrition panel done to identify any current nutritional deficiencies and take supplements to correct them.

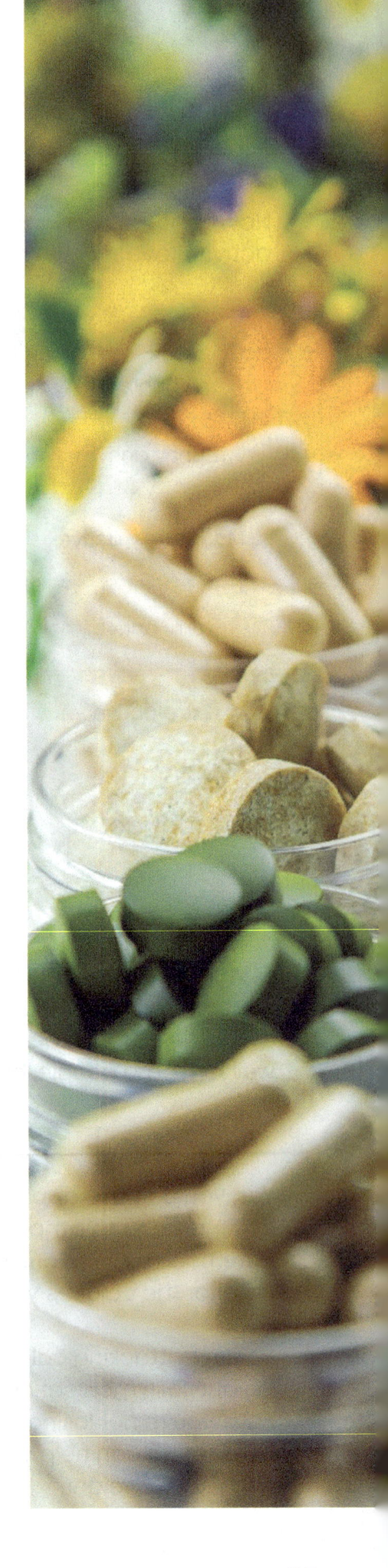

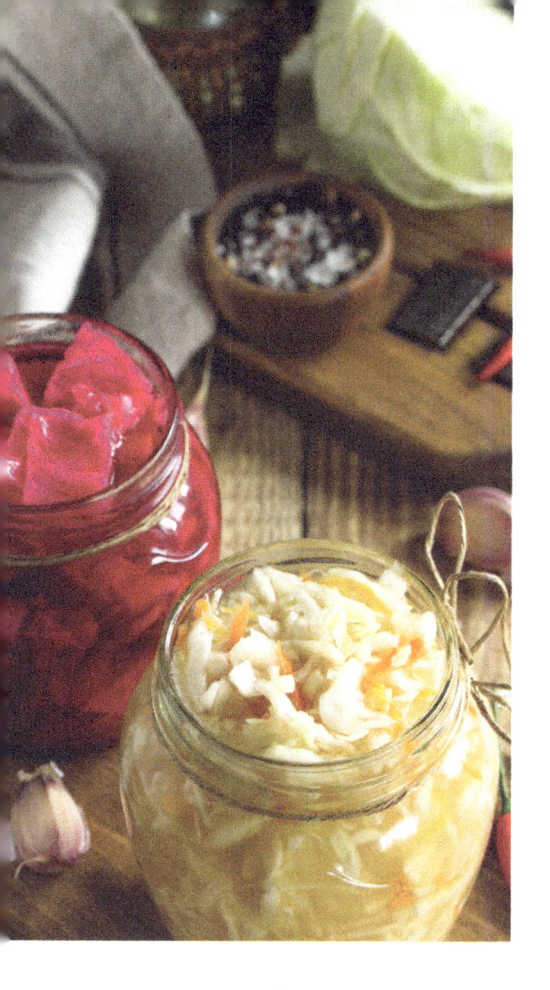

# Probiotics

The most common side effects of semaglutide are related to your GI tract. For this reason it makes sense to discuss with your doctor the use of probiotics while on this weight loss medication. Probiotics can help strengthen your GI system.

Taking probiotic supplements is the easiest way to consume the different types of probiotics that you need in sufficient quantities. However, adding probiotic foods to your diet can provide you with additional benefits.

**Foods high in probiotics**

- Yogurt
- Kefir
- Sauerkraut
- Tempeh
- Natto
- Kimchi
- Miso
- Kombucha
- Pickles
- Traditional buttermilk
- Fermented cheeses: swiss, provolone, gouda, cheddar, edam, gruyere, cottage cheese.

**Prebiotics can also be beneficial to improve your gut health but it is easier to get them from your diet.**

### Wondering what is the difference between prebiotics and probiotics?

Probiotics are live bacteria that support gut health. Prebiotics are non-digestible fibers in food that feed the good bacteria already in your gut. Probiotics add good bacteria, while prebiotics feed them, both working together to keep your gut healthy.

## Foods **rich in prebiotics:**

- Chicory root
- Dandelion greens
- Jerusalem artichoke
- Garlic
- Onions
- Leeks
- Asparagus
- Bananas (green, unripe)
- Barley
- Oats
- Apples
- Potatoes (cooked and cooled)
- Cocoa
- Konjac Root
- Burdock Root
- Flaxseeds
- Yacon Root
- Jicama Root
- Wheat Bran
- Seaweed

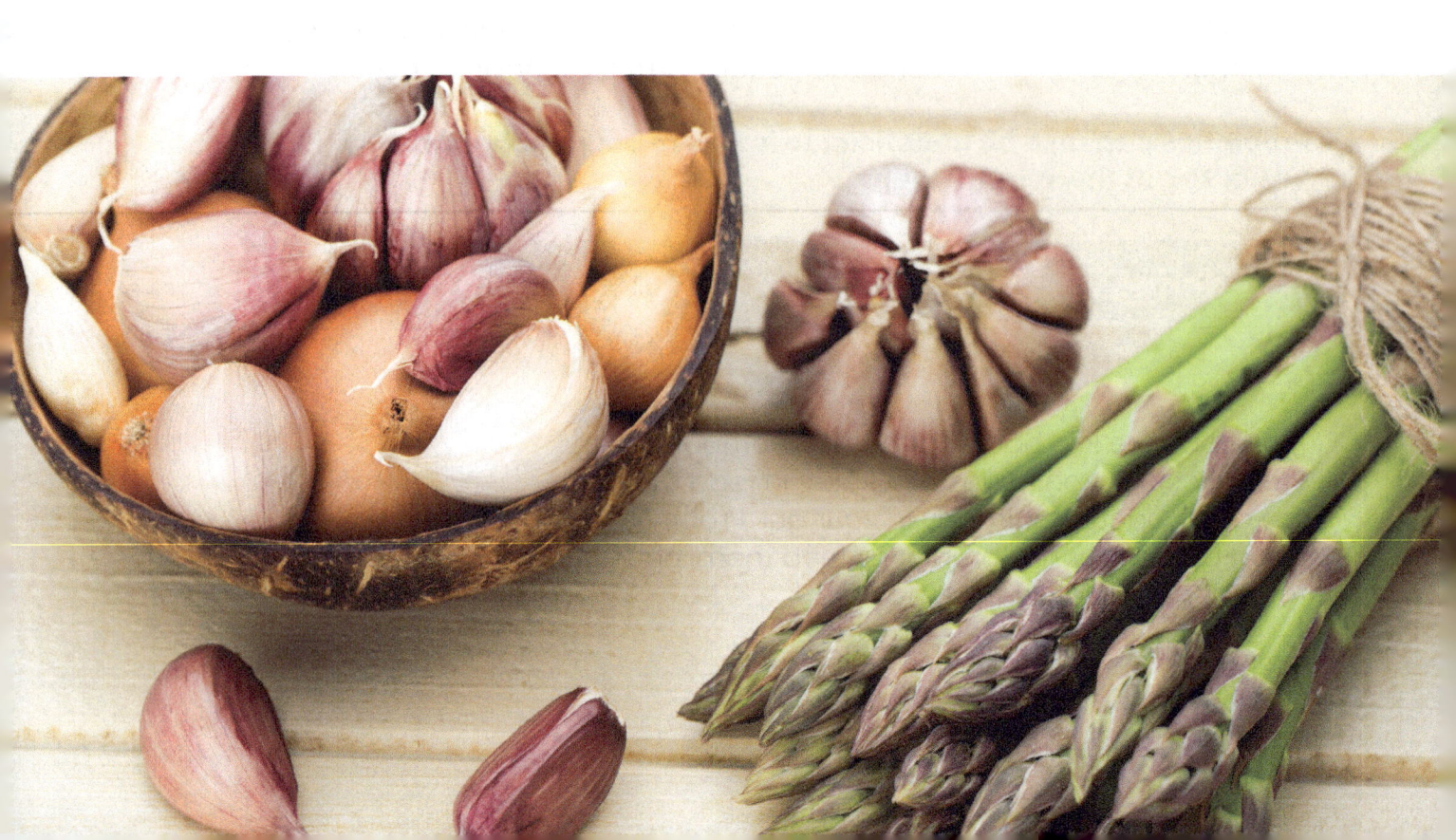

# Eating **out**

To maintain simplicity and consistency in your diet, you can apply the same principles even when dining out. Prioritize protein and vegetables as the focal point of your meal, ensuring they occupy a significant portion of your plate. Opt for carbohydrates only if they are an integral part of the meal (like in sushi) or indulge in small amounts to satisfy your palate.

However, it's important that you give yourself the flexibility to occasionally enjoy smaller portions of foods you love. By incorporating these practices, you're cultivating sustainable and healthy eating habits that accommodate both your nutritional needs and personal preferences.

After all, you are striving to create sustainable eating habits, and eating out is common for most people. When eating out, forget the all or nothing mentality. Just because you eat out doesn't mean you have to forget about your weight-loss journey.

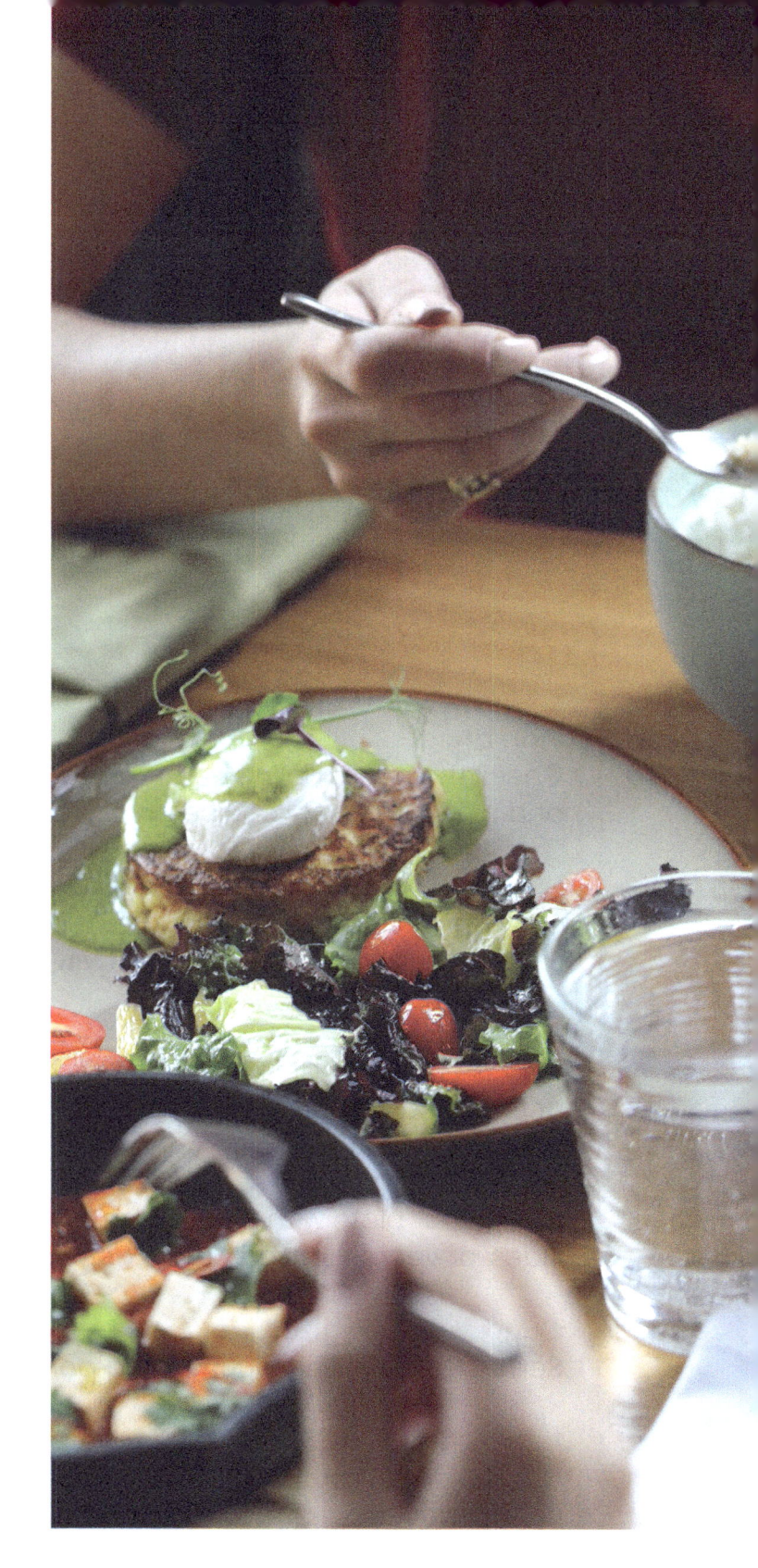

Copyright © 2024 by Dr. Su-Nui Escobar, RDN, LDN

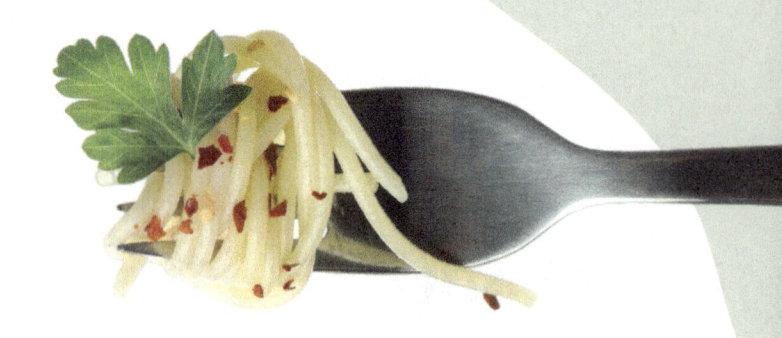

Regardless of what you eat, go back to your normal meal plan at the next meal.

## Tips for eating out

- **Plan ahead.**
  Check the menu online beforehand to identify healthier options and plan your meal choices in advance.

- **Look for grilled, steamed, or baked options.**
  Choose dishes that are prepared using healthier cooking methods rather than fried or heavily sauced items.

- **Opt for lean protein.**
  Choose dishes that feature lean proteins like grilled chicken, fish, or tofu, and ask for dressing or sauces on the side.

- **Load up on vegetables.**
  Fill up your plate with vegetables by choosing salads, vegetable sides, or veggie-based dishes as your main course.

- **Control portion sizes.**
  Semaglutide will help controlling portion size.

- **Limit alcohol and sugary drinks.**
  Opt for water, sparkling water, unsweetened tea, and other low-calorie beverages.

- **Be flexible.**
  Don't stress about finding the perfect healthy option every time you eat out. It's okay to indulge occasionally, just aim to make healthier choices most of the time.

# Semaglutide Side Effects (and How to Get Relief)

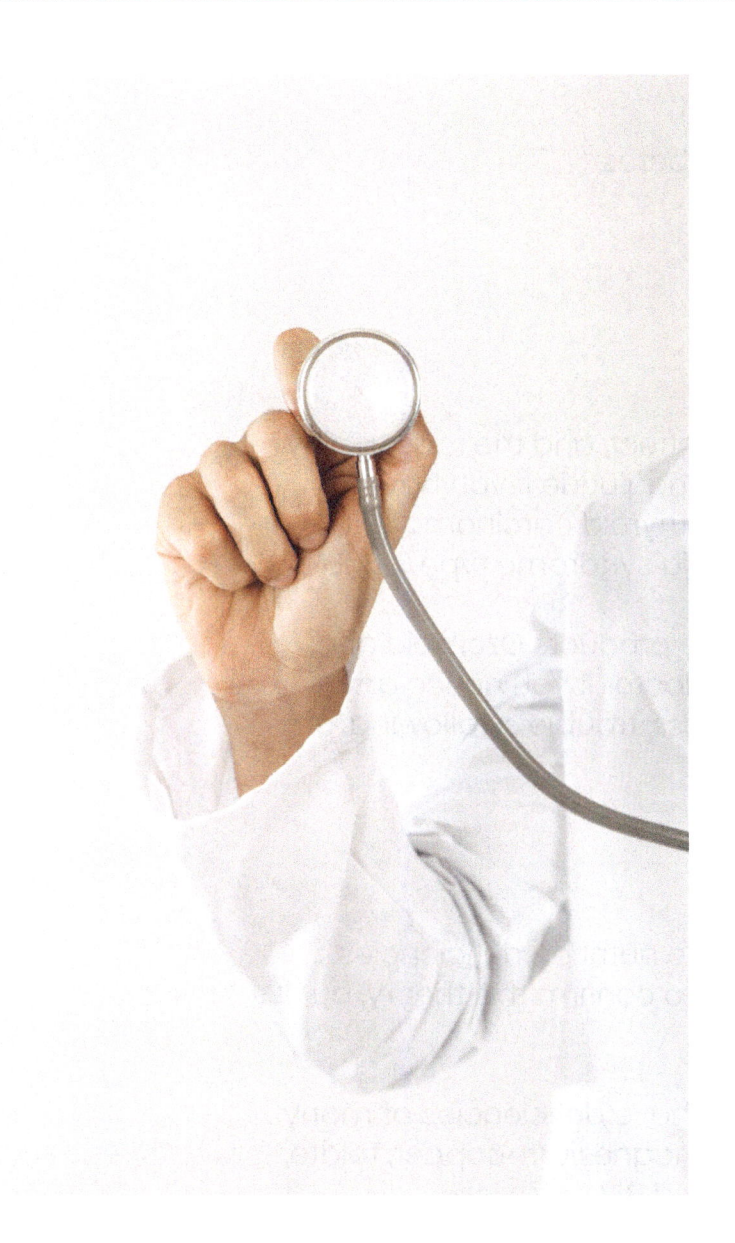

## Side Effects

Like any other medication, semaglutide has side effects. The most common ones are related to the medication's impact on the gastrointestinal tract (GI) and are temporary, meaning they go away after some time, once the body gets used to the medication.

Side effects are the reason why semaglutide starts at a lower dose and escalates over time.

**Common side effects of semaglutide include:**

- Constipation
- Diarrhea
- Nausea
- Vomiting
- Burping
- Stomach pain
- Bloating
- Fatigue
- Headache
- Dizziness

Diet, physical activity, and lifestyle can help minimize some of these symptoms.

**Rare but serious side effects include:**

- Pancreatitis
- Gallbladder issues
- Hypoglycemia, especially if paired with a blood glucose lowering medication
- Kidney problems
- Allergic reactions
- Changes in vision in people with diabetes
- Increase heart rate
- Depression and suicidal thoughts

**Black Box Warnings**

Thyroid cancer is another serious side effect, and the reason why your doctor is not likely to prescribe semaglutide if you have a family or personal history of medullary thyroid carcinoma (MCT) or if you have multiple endocrine neoplasia syndrome type 2 (MEN 2).

Novo, the manufacturer of semaglutide products Ozempic and Wegovy, recommends talking to your doctor if you notice any lump or swelling in your neck, hoarseness, trouble swallowing, or shortness of breath.

**Nutrition Deficiencies**

Other potential side effects may include nutrition deficiencies. Currently there is insufficient research to confirm this theory, but it's a good idea to consider the possibility.

It's known that obese individuals often have deficiencies of many nutrients including iron, zinc, calcium, magnesium, copper, folate, potassium, selenium, and vitamins A and B12.

These deficiencies can worsen after starting semaglutide, as people eat less and often not enough. However, because this drug is relatively new, more research is needed to confirm this potential side effect.

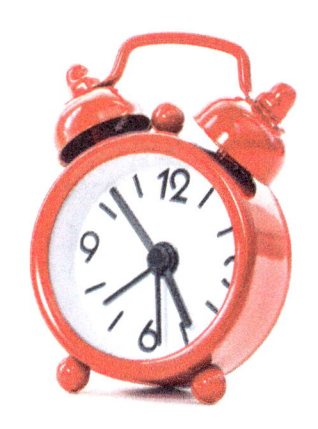

## How Long do Side Effects Last?

According to research, symptoms are transitory, meaning they last for a few days or a few weeks while the body gets used to the medication.

Often, symptoms worsen a day or two after taking the medication but then gradually improve over the following days. It's also common to see that symptoms appear or worsen in the first week or two after starting a new dose.

**It's always a good idea to keep your prescribing doctor aware of any symptoms you are experiencing on the medication.** But if your symptoms are severe or interfering with your daily activities, call your doctor immediately.

# Constipation

Constipation is a very common side effect of this obesity medication. You can expect changes in your bowel movements, that's normal. But to clarify, constipation is defined as having difficulty passing stools or having fewer than three bowel movements a week.

Here's how this medication may contribute to constipation:

- **Slows digestion:**
  This helps with weight loss as you feel full for a longer period of time. However, it results in constipation and other GI symptoms.

- **Reduced intestinal motility:**
  In other words, it reduces the action of the muscles in your GI system that help the food pass through your body.

- **Decrease in dietary fiber:**
  You eat less overall, including those foodsn that are high in fiber.

- **Decrease in fluid intake:**
  You might not feel thirsty, which results in harder and drier stools.

**Essential Tips for Easing Constipation**

- **Increase your fiber intake:**
  Fiber is essential to improve digestion. It adds bulk to your stool and helps it pass through your digestive system more easily.

- **Drink plenty of fluids:**
  Staying hydrated is crucial for maintaining regular bowel movements. Fluids help soften the stool and make it easier to pass.

- **Physical activity:**
  Engaging in physical activity stimulates the muscles in your intestines, promoting bowel movements.

Once you cover the basic nutrition and lifestyle changes to relieve constipation, there are many other things you can try. But always start with these three basic diet and lifestyle changes.

## Foods That **Relieve Constipation**

Some foods are amazing at relieving constipation—worth trying!

- **Prune juice:**
  This juice is so helpful that many hospitals keep it in stock to help with constipation. The power is in the sorbitol these fruits contain, which helps soften stool and stimulates bowel movements. Try drinking 4 to 6 ounces of unsweetened prune juice in the mornings.

- **Coffee:**
  Yes, you read correctly—coffee can help with constipation by stimulating the digestive system. The caffeine in coffee acts as a natural laxative, encouraging bowel movements. Enjoy a cup of coffee to help get things moving.

- **Olive oil:**
  Olive oil helps your stools to pass by lubricating your intestines. For best results, try taking a teaspoon of extra-virgin olive oil on an empty stomach. You can also drizzle it over salads or use it to top hummus or cooked veggies. No need to stress—it won't throw off your weight-loss journey in such small amounts.

**Additional Nutrition and Lifestyle Tips to Improve Constipation**

- **Avoid meals high in fat.**
  Fat takes longer to digest, so avoiding high-fat food can help with constipation. Examples include fried foods, baked goods (such as pastries), and fast food.

- **Establish a regular bathroom routine.**
  Set aside specific times during the day to use the bathroom. This can help regulate your body's natural rhythm and train your bowels to have more regularity.

- **Avoid delaying bowel movements.**
  When you feel the urge to have a bowel movement, try not to postpone it. Ignoring the urge can make your stool become harder and more difficult to pass.

- **Use a squatting stool.**
  Also known as poop stools, a squatting stool can help you position your body in a way that makes it easier to push waste.

**Over-The-Counter Remedies**

There are many over-the-counter remedies for constipation. Here is a list of the different types to help you understand them better. Which one is the best for you? Reach out to your prescribing physician to figure out what works best for your symptoms.

- **Bulk formers:**
  These add some extra bulk to your stool, making it easy for your gut to push it all along.

- **Stool softeners:**
  They soak up water like a sponge, making your stool softer and gentler on the way out.

- **Oral stimulants:**
  Need a little push? Oral stimulants give your intestines a nudge in the right direction.

- **Oral osmotics.**
  These pull water into the mix, softening up your stools for easier passage.

## When to Call Your Doctor

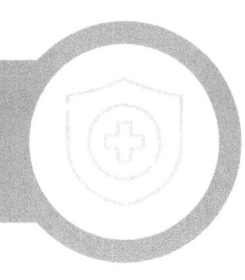

Changes in bowel movements are common while taking semaglutide, but it's important to **inform your doctor** when you notice them.

If natural remedies don't provide relief, discuss it with your physician to identify the best medication for constipation or adjust the dosage of semaglutide if constipation becomes troublesome.

Additionally, severe constipation—especially if accompanied by abdominal pain—could indicate a more serious medical issue, so **it's wise not to ignore it.**

# Diarrhea

Diarrhea is another common symptom of semaglutide for weight loss. It's caused by the effect of this medication on the gut and is more likely at higher doses.

Now, this is the interesting part of semaglutide diarrhea—it can happen to people with chronic constipation. When you have constipation, the old stool becomes hard, doesn't move, and blocks the colon. Then as new stool forms, the blocked colon cannot absorb the water from the old stool. So, the new stools leak around the old stool. This is called overflow diarrhea. This is the reason why you will benefit from speaking to your doctor to determine the best way to treat diarrhea.

Before talking about how to control diarrhea, let's mention the importance of drinking enough fluids to prevent dehydration.

Diarrhea can cause your body to lose a lot of fluids and electrolytes quickly, leading to dehydration. By drinking water, you can replenish the fluids lost through diarrhea and maintain hydration.

Now that we covered that, let's move to **natural remedies.**

## **Changes** in Your Diet

- **Avoid foods high in fat.**
  High-fat foods can worsen diarrhea for several reasons. Firstly, excess fat can break down in the colon, leading to the release of additional fluid and resulting in loose stool. Additionally, high-fat foods might not be absorbed properly, further contributing to digestive issues.

- **Avoid sugary drinks.**
  Sugar stimulates the gut and as a response, the gut secretes more water and electrolytes, which loosen stools.

- **Limit or avoid sugar alcohols.**
  Sugar alcohol is known for causing upset stomachs in certain individuals. They are often found in sugar-free foods.

- **Avoid spicy foods.**
Spicy foods contain compounds that can irritate your GI tract, worsening diarrhea in some people. Additionally, spicy foods may exacerbate other GI conditions, further contributing to diarrhea symptoms.

- **Eat bland foods.**
Foods such as rice, applesauce, bananas, chicken, and toast are well tolerated. Start slowly, and incorporate other foods once you start feeling better.

**Over-the-Counter Medications**

Before taking over-the-counter medications, talk to your healthcare provider to determine what is best for you.

## When to Call Your Doctor

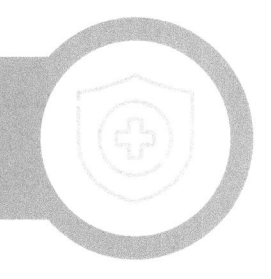

Contact your healthcare provider if:

- Diarrhea lasts more than 2 days
- You experience excessive thirst, dry mouth or skin, lack of urination, severe weakness, or dizziness
- Severe abdominal or rectal pain
- You have bloody or dark stools
- You have a fever

# Nausea

Nausea is another common side effect of this medication. Often, both of these side effects worsen as the dose increases and during the first or second day after the injection. However, there are a few things you can do to feel better.

## Changes in Your Diet

- **Eat small, frequent meals.**
  Nausea could be related to slow digestion. Instead of having large meals, opt for smaller, more frequent meals throughout the day. This will prevent your stomach from becoming too full, which can trigger nausea.

- **Avoid triggering foods and smells.**
  Certain food, strong smells, or cooking odors can exacerbate nausea. Identify any specific triggers for you and avoid them as much as possible.

- **Avoid fried foods.**
  Foods that are high in fat are more difficult to digest. So, stick to lighter, low-fat foods.

- **Avoid spicy or heavily seasoned foods.**
  Opt for plain dishes, as heavily seasoned and spicy foods might further irritate the stomach.

- **Eat slowly.**
  Take your time when eating, and chew your food thoroughly to aid digestion.

- **Stay upright after eating.**
  Avoid lying down immediately after eating, as that can worsen this symptom.

**Natural Remedies to Relieve Nausea**

- **Ginger.**
  Ginger has natural anti-nausea properties. You can try ginger tea, ginger ale, ginger candies, or even chewing on a small piece of fresh ginger to help alleviate nausea. You can also buy ginger chews or drops designed for nausea relief at your local pharmacy or an online retailer.

- **Peppermint.**
  Peppermint is known for its soothing effect on the stomach. Sip on peppermint tea or suck on peppermint candies to help calm nausea.

- **Lemon.**
  Lemon's smell and its tangy acidity can help ease nausea. Simply take a whiff of a freshly sliced lemon or squeeze some lemon juice into your water or tea for a refreshing remedy.

- **Fresh air.**
  If you're feeling nauseous, try going outside for some fresh air or opening a window. Fresh air and good ventilation can help reduce feelings of queasiness.

- **Stay hydrated.**
  Sip on clear fluids like water, herbal tea, or electrolyte-rich drinks to prevent dehydration. Take small, frequent sips to avoid overwhelming your stomach.

## Foods That are **Easier to Tolerate**

When you are nauseous, there are a few foods that are easier for your stomach to tolerate.

- **High-protein diet.**
  Foods that are high in protein are less likely to worsen this side effect when compared to a diet that is high in carbohydrates.

- **Foods served cold or at room temperature.**
  Cold or room-temperature foods are easier to handle because they have milder smells and flavors which are less likely to trigger nausea.

- **Liquid foods.**
  If solid foods are difficult to tolerate, consider eating soft or liquid options, like smoothies, soups, yogurt, or applesauce until your nausea improves. I usually recommend choosing foods that are high in protein, like Greek yogurt and smoothies made with protein powder or nut butter.

**Other Helpful Tips**

If you find yourself with worse nausea the day or two after the medication, prepare for it in advance. Take your injections when you have time to rest. Also, have easy-to-tolerate foods available for those days.

## When to Call Your Doctor

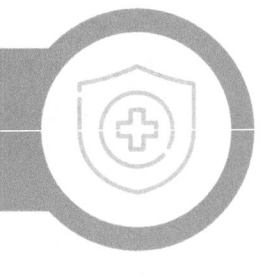

Talk to your doctor if nausea persists, if you are vomiting, or if it's interfering with your daily life.

If you cannot eat due to nausea or vomiting, **call your doctor if it persists for more than 2 days**. Also, mention this symptom to your physician or healthcare provider.

# Burping

Semaglutide can cause some people to have sulfur burps, and the taste of these burps likely resembles rotten eggs.

Sulfur burps can happen likely because of the slow digestion caused by semaglutide. The longer food is in your stomach, the more likely it is to produce gas that has to leave the body.

Luckily, burping or belching is not a common symptom but it happens.

## Tips to Ease **Sulfur Burps**

**Changes in Your Diet**

Reduce foods that cause excessive burping and foods that are high in sulfur. However, it is essential to find a good balance to avoid cutting important foods from your diet, such as protein.

**Foods that cause excessive burping:**

- Legumes and beans
- Cruciferous vegetables such as broccoli, cabbage, Brussels sprouts, and cauliflower.
- Beer and wine
- Dairy foods

**Foods that are high in sulfur**

- Garlic, onions, leeks, and scallions
- Foods high in protein
- Nuts
- Condiments and spices sharp in flavor such as horseradish, mustard, curry powder, and ground ginger

Other diet changes you can make include:

- **Avoid carbonated beverages.** These drinks can exacerbate gas and result in worse-smelling/tasting burps.

- **Avoid excess sugar.** Limiting sugar intake can reduce burps, as sugar feeds the bacteria that produce hydrogen sulfide.

- **Drink less alcohol.** Reducing alcohol can decrease burps and improve digestion, which can help. Because this unwanted side effect is likely caused by slow digestion, improving digestion is a good step to decrease sulfur burps.

## When to See a Doctor

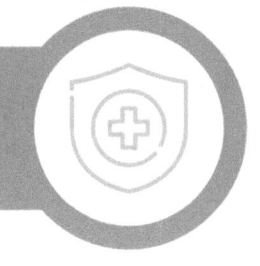

Call your healthcare provider if sulfur burps do not improve after a few weeks or if you also have abdominal pain, severe constipation or vomiting.

Also call if they are impacting your life.

# Fatigue

There can be several reasons why semaglutide causes fatigue. The medication itself might cause fatigue, but one big reason you might feel tired when taking it is that you're not eating enough.

I understand that you want to lose weight as fast as possible, but eating at least 1200 calories if you are female and 1500 calories if you are a male is crucial for good health.

So, make sure you eat at least three meals or two meals and a snack a day and make every meal count.

Iron-deficiency anemia is another possible cause of fatigue—especially if you're eating less animal protein or other foods high in iron such as legumes, dark leafy greens, and iron-fortified foods.

Also, if you notice that your fatigue is worse after the injection, schedule your medication right before you have time to rest. For many people, this means injecting on Friday night, and planning to rest the next day.

# Other Common Concerns

# Not Eating Enough

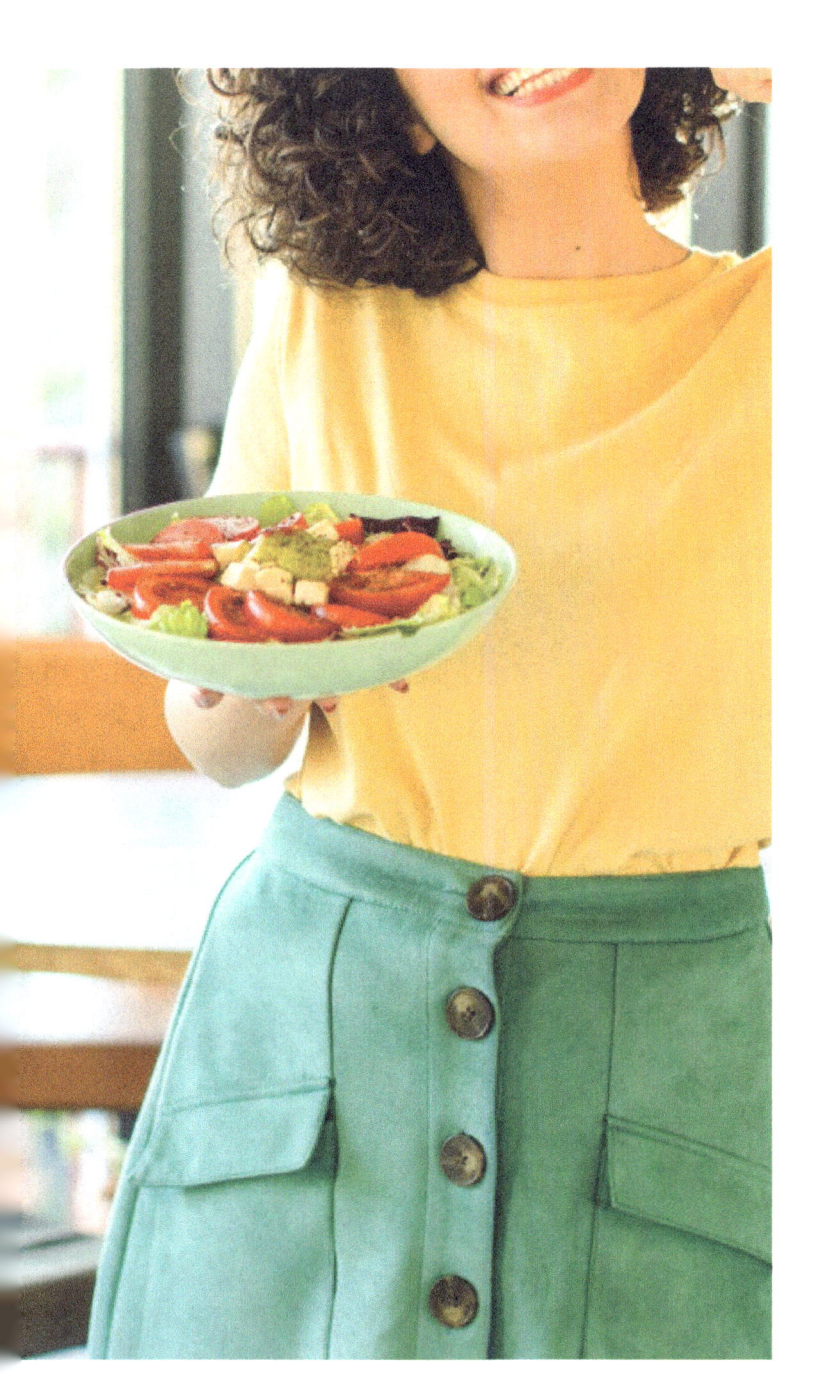

Amazingly, eating too little is a possibility while taking semaglutide. Of course, you want to create a calorie deficit and lose weight, but there is actually such a thing as eating too little.

**Not eating enough can cause serious nutritional deficiencies and create a range of health issues.**

If you are a woman, aim to eat at least 1,200 calories per day. If you are a man, aim for at least 1,500. However, these calorie levels might not be enough if you started your weight loss journey with a BMI of over 35m/kg2.

If you're having difficulty eating enough, ensure you consume enough nutrition by focusing on nutrient-dense foods like protein, dark green leafy vegetables, and nuts. In other words, **make every bite count.**

## Tips: Eat Enough

1. Aim to eat at least two meals and one snack per day.

2. Drink a protein shake instead of a meal when you don't feel hungry. Add a piece of fruit to the shake, if possible, or eat some fruit along with the shake.

3. Add cheese or eggs to meals for extra protein and calories.

4. Top salads, soups, and other dishes with seeds such as sunflower or pumpkin for added flavor and texture.

5. Drink smoothies made with fruit like bananas that are higher in calories than other fruit choices.

6. Consume snacks between meals such as nut bars or yogurt parfaits that can help increase caloric intake without taking up too much volume at mealtime.

7. Include calorie-dense whole grains like oats or quinoa into breakfast bowls for an additional boost of energy throughout the day.

8. Avoid foods that make you feel full without providing nutrients, such as fast food.

9. Be mindful of how much you eat. It is easy to skip meals on semaglutide as you might not feel hungry.

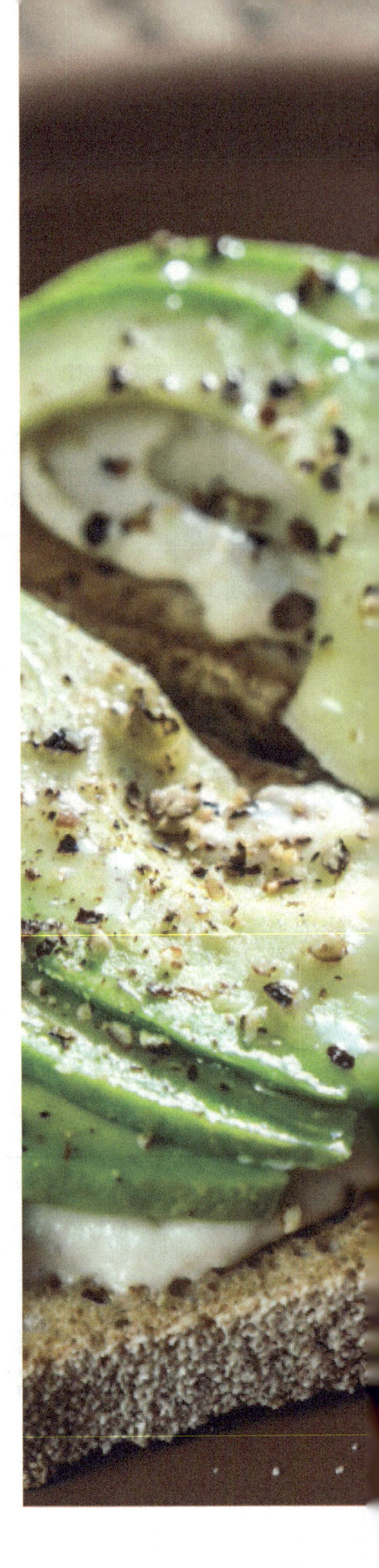

# **Not** Losing Weight

Let's start by setting realistic expectations.

In clinical trials, people taking semaglutide lose an average of approximately 15% of their initial body weight over 68 weeks (Steps 1 and Step 5 studies). This means that if you start your weight around 250 pounds, you can expect to lose an average of 37 pounds over a year. Thus losing 1-2 pounds a week is very reasonable. The best part of using semaglutide is that weight loss is consistent and you can see a significant difference over time.

Of course, many people lose more than the average weight and some people will lose less.

Also, it's important to understand that weight loss is not achieved in a straight line. Often people plateau for a few days or a few weeks.

If you're not losing weight, there are a few things you need to check.

- Are you following a healthy eating plan?
- Are your portions a reasonable size or extra-large?
- Are you eating high-calorie foods?
- Are you consuming a lot of calories in beverages?
- Are you exercising enough?
- Are you sleeping at least 7 hours most nights?
- Do you have unrealistic expectations about your weight loss?

The answer to these questions can give you an insight into what to do next.

# Possible Reasons Why You Are Not Losing Weight

Let's go over the potential causes and the solutions.

- **Dose is low.**
  People respond differently to the medication. Some start losing weight as soon as they start the medication, even at the lowest dose. Others don't lose significant weight until they reach the maximum dose. If you're in the earlier doses of the medication, it might be a matter of time.

- **Inconsistent use.**
  You must inject semaglutide once a week on the same day of the week. Inconsistent use can slow down weight loss.

- **You are not following a healthy eating plan.**
  You may be eating small amounts of the wrong foods. If you are relying mostly on the medication but not following a plan, it is time to focus on healthy eating. Just follow the plan outlined in this guide.

- **You are eating too many calories.**
  Sometimes it is easy to realize when you are eating too many calories, but other times you need to closely examine what you eat. If you are in doubt, I suggest you track your calories using an app and adjust your food to meet your calorie needs.

- **You are drinking your calories.**
  Drinks can pack a large number of calories. So be mindful about how many sugary drinks and alcohol you are drinking.

- **You are not eating enough protein.**
  Protein can help you feel fuller for longer, decreasing the chance of overeating or snacking between meals. Additionally, it aids in controlling appetite and satiety.

- **Lack of physical activity.**
  Many people find that at the beginning, semaglutide does the trick, but as time passes, they need to start exercising to lose weight. The goal is to exercise moderately at least 150 minutes a week—or 75 minutes of intense physical activity. It's also important to add strength training 2 to 3 times a week.

# Move **More**

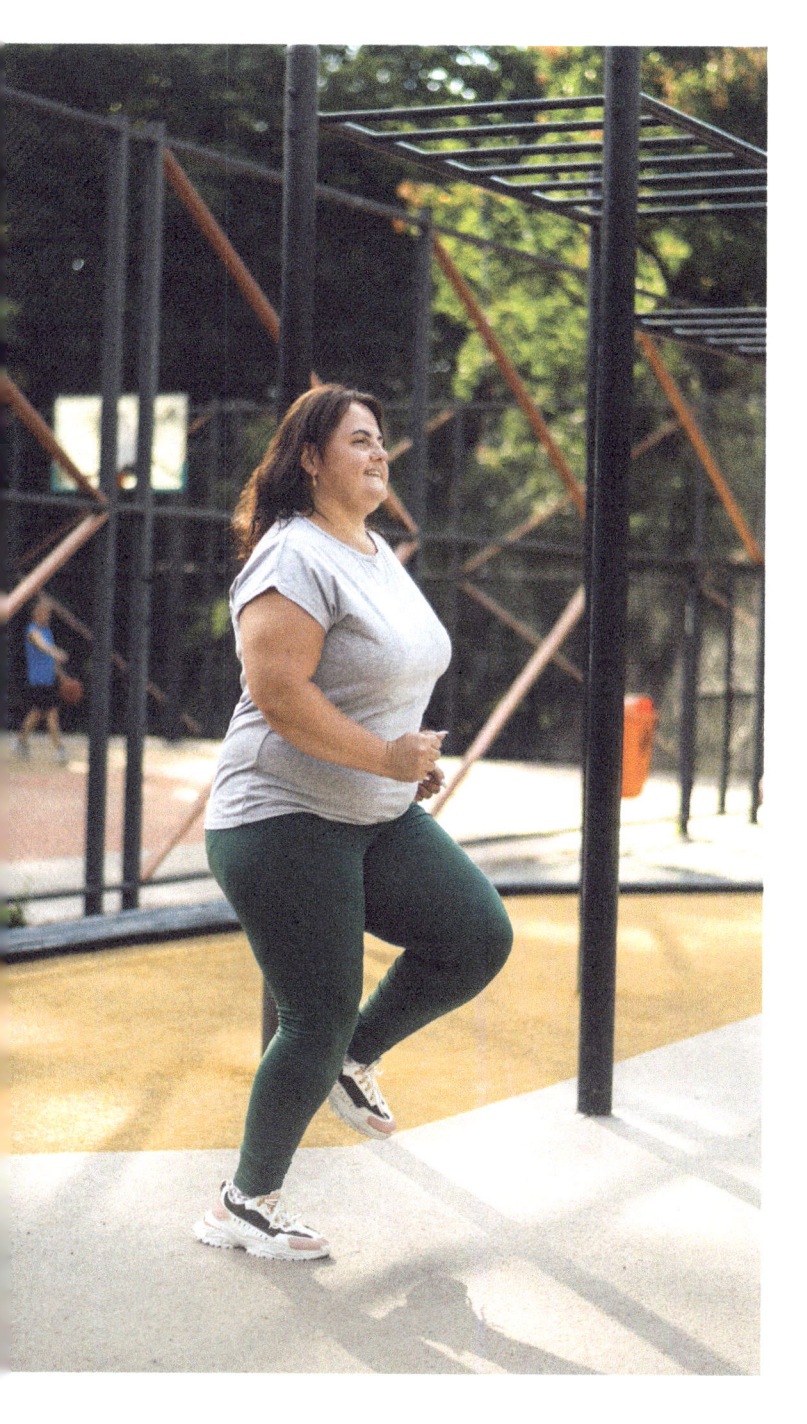

While physical activity is not the focus of this book, it's important to mention a few important things.

First, there are many reasons why physical activity is recommended while taking semaglutide. However, we will focus on the following ones:

1. Optimizes weight loss
2. Tones the body
3. Maintains muscle mass
4. Optimizes your metabolism
5. Minimizes side effects

## How Much Exercise Do You Need?

The U.S. Department of Health and Human Services recommends that you exercise for at least 150 minutes of moderate aerobic physical activity or 75 minutes of vigorous activity.

In addition, you will benefit from doing strength training exercises for all the major muscle groups at least two times a week. Lastly, adding flexibility to this routine can prevent injuries.

### Cardiovascular Exercises

Cardio is essential for weight loss and overall health. It helps you lose weight by burning calories. Plus, this type of exercise boosts your metabolism, making it easier to keep the weight off. But it's not just about weight loss—cardio also lowers the risk of heart disease, diabetes, and stroke.

Doing cardiovascular exercise even improves your mood, reduces stress, and helps you sleep better—all of which can also help with weight loss.

So, adding cardio to your routine can help optimize your weight loss while on semaglutide, but also it's great for feeling amazing overall.

**Examples of aerobic exercise:**

- Dance videos
- Walking
- Running or jogging
- Cycling
- Swimming
- Jumping rope
- Dancing
- Kickboxing
- Rowing
- Elliptical machine
- Hiking
- Cardio circuit training
- High-intensity interval training (HIIT)
- Water aerobics

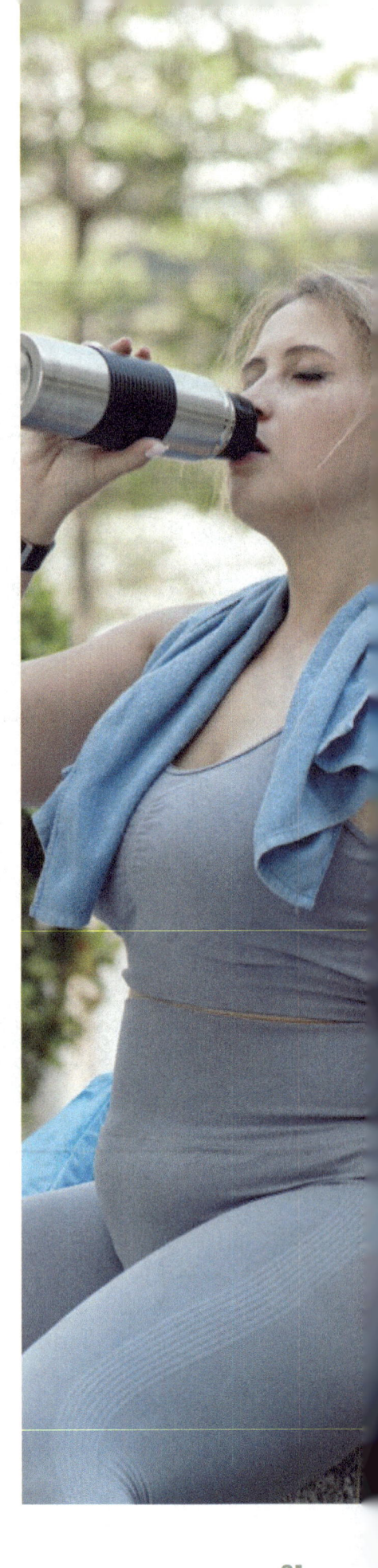

For maximum efficacy, make sure that you perform the activity at an intensity that challenges you.

A common question I get is whether walking is enough. Honestly, walking is an amazing start—especially if you're not used to exercising—but in order to get the best of cardio, you need to make it challenging, and for most people, walking is generally not challenging exercise.

## Strength Training

This is a must while taking weight loss medication.

It's totally normal to lose both fat and muscle as you lose weight. But if you want to optimize your weight loss and achieve a toned, healthy look, it's important to maintain as much muscle as possible. To do this, you need to work out your muscles.

There's really no way around it! Especially if you are over the age of 30, as you naturally start losing muscle around this time.

**Example of strength training exercises:**

- Bodyweight exercises
- Free weights
- Resistance bands
- Functional training
- Plyometric exercises
- Power yoga
- Pilates

## Flexibility

It is always a good idea to stretch your muscles to prevent injuries. Flexibility exercises play a crucial role in maintaining joint mobility and preventing muscle tightness.

By regularly incorporating stretching into your routine, you can improve your range of motion, enhance flexibility, and reduce the risk of strains, sprains, and other injuries during physical activity.

## Tips for **Incorporating Physical Activity**

The following tips can help you get started. However, select only the ones that make sense for you.

- **Start small.**
  Begin with a short burst of activity, like a 10-minute walk, and gradually increase the length and/or intensity as you feel comfortable.

- **Find what you love.**
  Choose activities you enjoy, whether it's dancing, hiking, or playing a sport, to make staying active more enjoyable.

- **Make it social.**
  Invite friends or family to join you for a walk, bike ride, or fitness class. Or join a gym and find your tribe there!

- **Set goals.**
  Set achievable goals, like walking a certain number of steps a day, or completing a workout session, to keep you motivated.

- **Be flexible.**
  Don't worry if you miss a workout or can't stick to your routine—just get back on track the next day and keep moving forward.

- **Mix it up.**
  Keep things interesting by trying different activities and workouts to prevent boredom and challenge your body in new ways.

- **Sneak in physical activity.**
  Look for opportunities to be active throughout your day, like taking the stairs instead of the elevator or doing squats while brushing your teeth.

- **Listen to your body.**
  Pay attention to how you feel during and after exercise, and adjust your intensity or duration accordingly to avoid injury and stay consistent.

# Mindful Eating

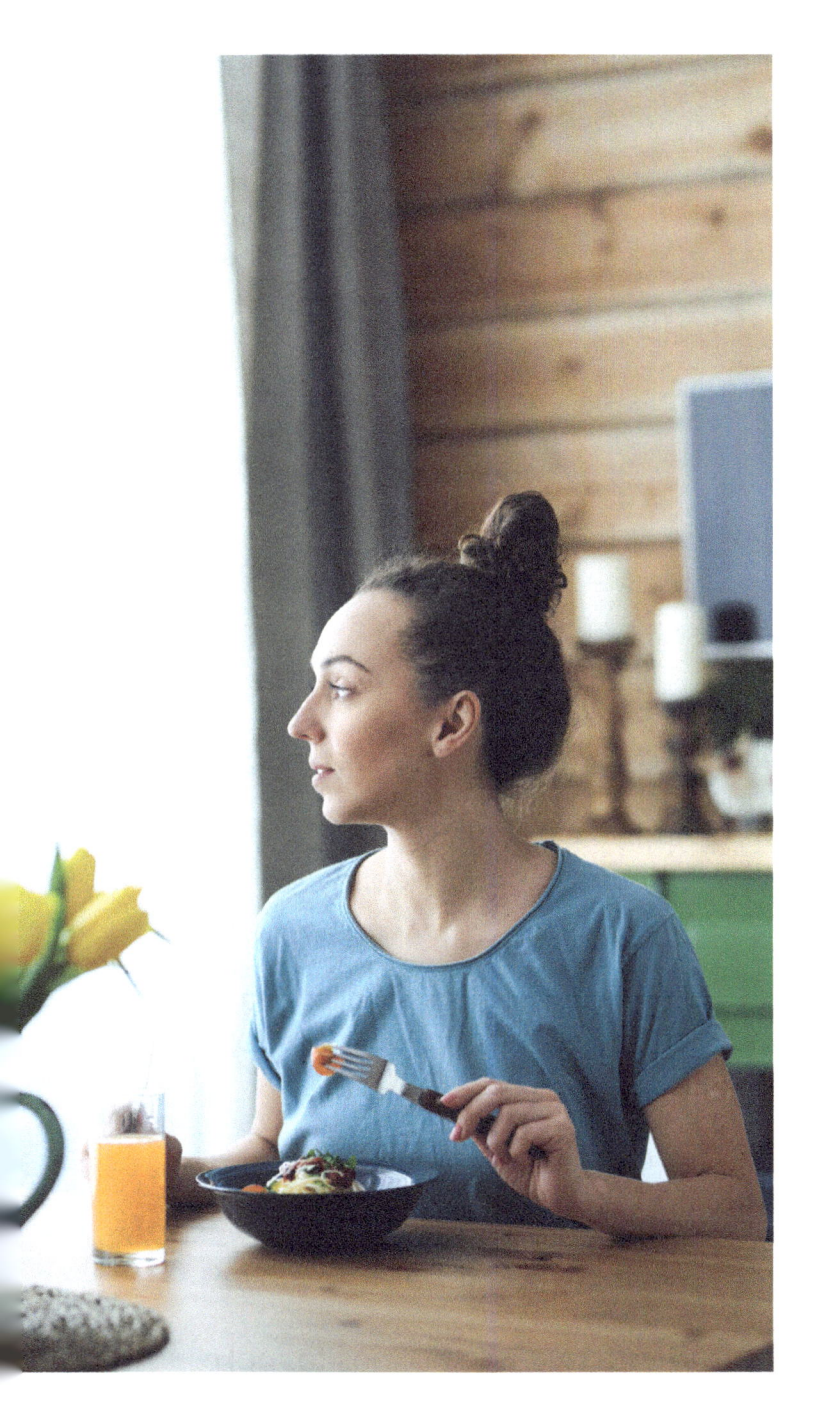

Mindful eating is the perfect complement to semaglutide and can help you reshape your relationship with food. With reduced anxiety around eating, it's now much easier to tune into internal hunger and satiety cues and understand the triggers that influence your eating behaviors.

By being mindful of all cues that impact eating behaviors and health, this technique becomes a valuable strategy for guiding food choices, optimizing health, and achieving a healthy weight.

### What is Mindful Eating?

Mindful eating is a practice that involves paying **full attention to the experience of eating and drinking**. It involves being present in the moment while eating, noticing the colors, smell, flavors, and textures of food, as well as the sensations within the body.

This practice also involves being aware of the emotions and thoughts that arise during eating, without judgment or criticism. The goal of mindful eating is to develop a more balanced and healthy relationship with food, free from the influences of external distractions, emotional eating, and unconscious habits. It encourages greater awareness of food choices, promotes enjoyment of eating, and supports overall well-being.

## **Benefits** of Mindful Eating

- Improves diet quality
- Better food choices
- Enhanced weight management
- Aids with disordered eating patterns
- Can help with emotional eating

## Mindful Eating **Checklist**

**AT THE BEGINNING OF THE WEEK:**

Prepare to make mindful food choices based on your preferences, health goals, and life events. Keep these tips in mind:

- Use the food list provided in this book to help you make healthy choices that you love.

- Create a simple meal plan to guide your grocery shopping, allowing flexibility for changes or new meal ideas. This book provides you with many recipes to give you ideas.

- Choose foods that align with your nutrition goals and your personal preferences.

  Be open to trying new foods to discover healthy options that you love.

- Keep your home and workplace stocked with nutrition options to make healthy eating more convenient and accessible.

## BEFORE YOUR MEALS:

Create an internal and external environment that enables you to focus on eating mindfully. By doing so you can be fully present and become aware of what you are eating.

**External environment:**

- Allow yourself time to eat
- Turn off all electronic devices
- Sit down
- Remove clutter from your table

**Internal environment:**

- Forget the all-or-nothing mentality, guilt, or any judgments about foods or yourself.
- Listen to your body and identify your hunger levels before you eat.

As you stop mindless eating, you will move effortlessly to an eating pattern that nourishes your body and your soul.

## AS YOU EAT:

- Eat slowly and pay attention to the flavor, texture, and smell of your food. **Be present.**
- Enjoy every bite of food.

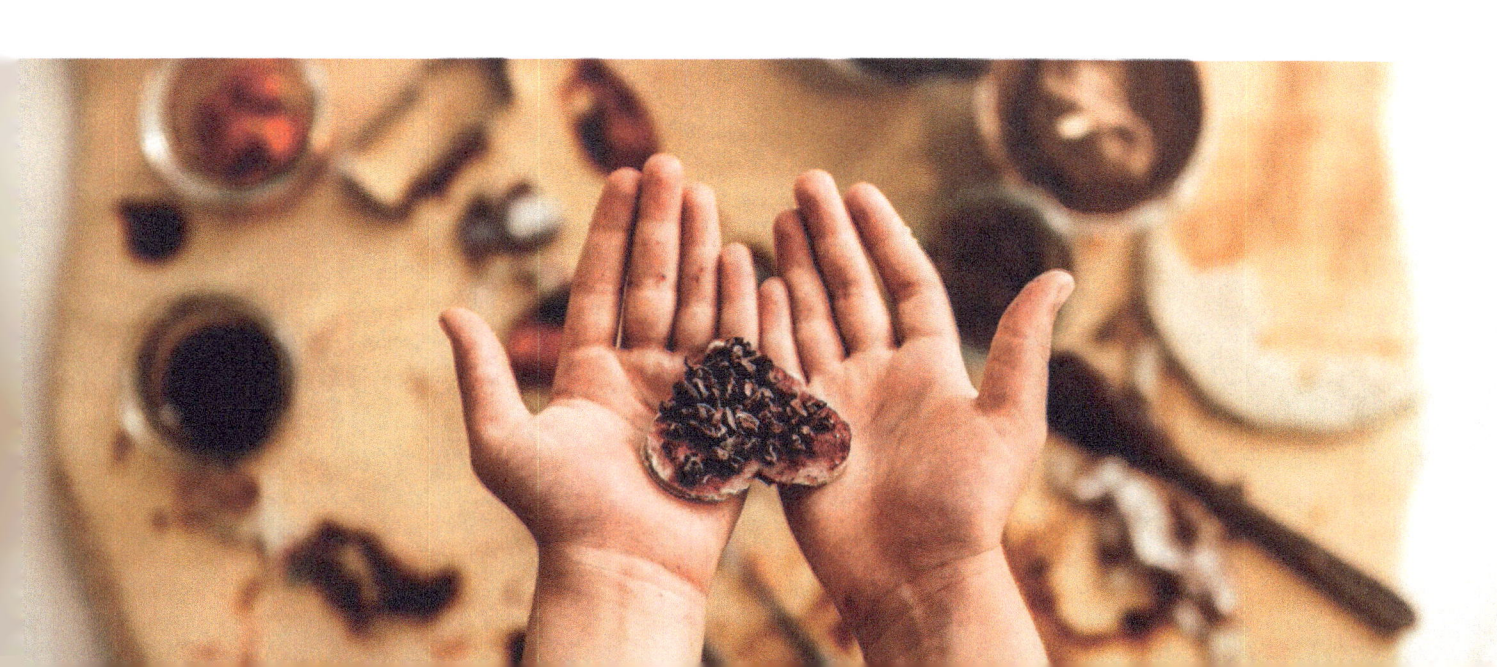

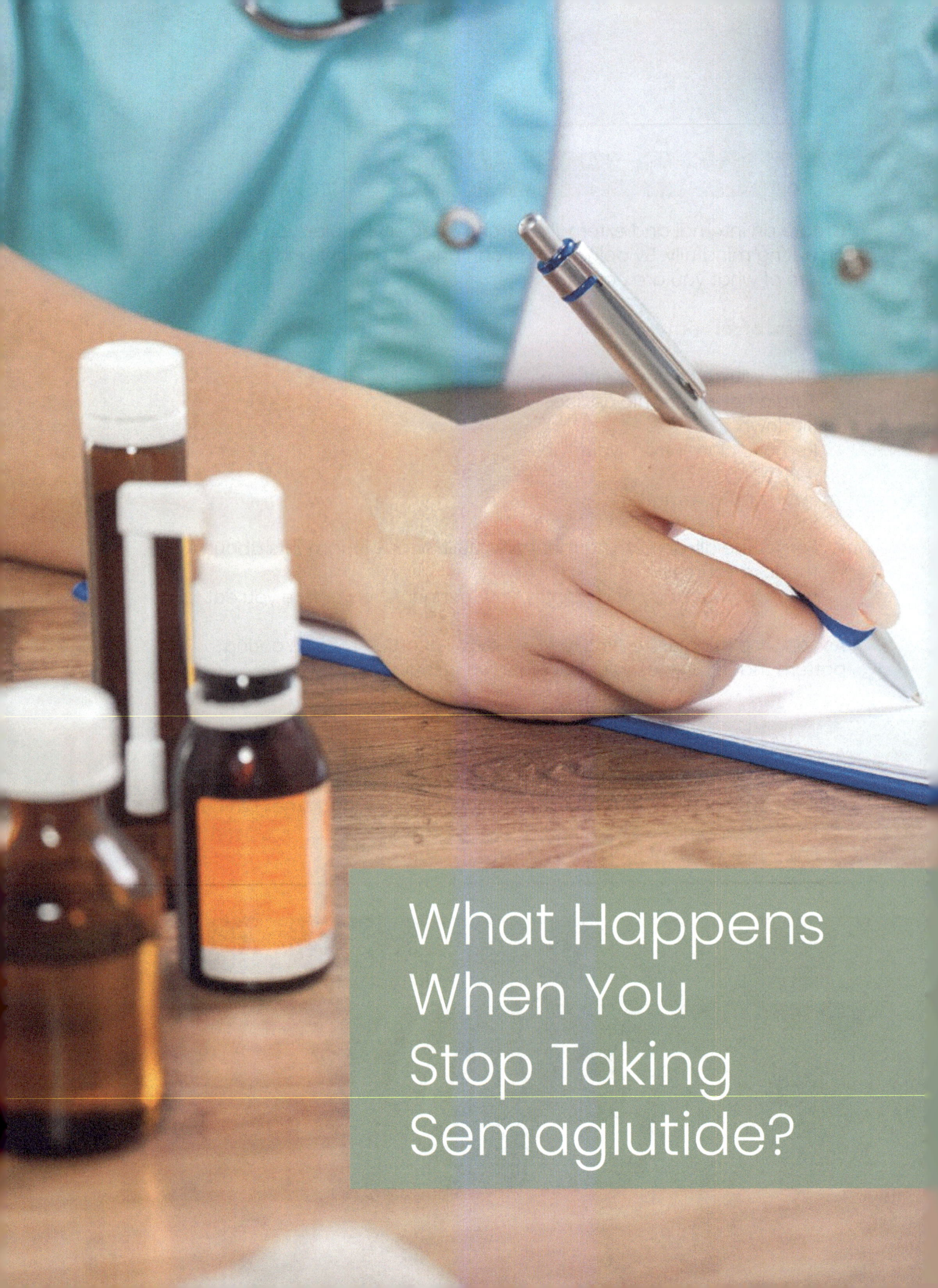

# What Happens When You Stop Taking Semaglutide?

If you decide—or need—to stop taking semaglutide, the effects of the medication will wear off and **you may start gaining back some of the weight you lost.**

In clinical trials, people who stopped taking semaglutide began to regain weight gradually. This is because you will start feeling hungry again, you will eat more and regain weight as a result.

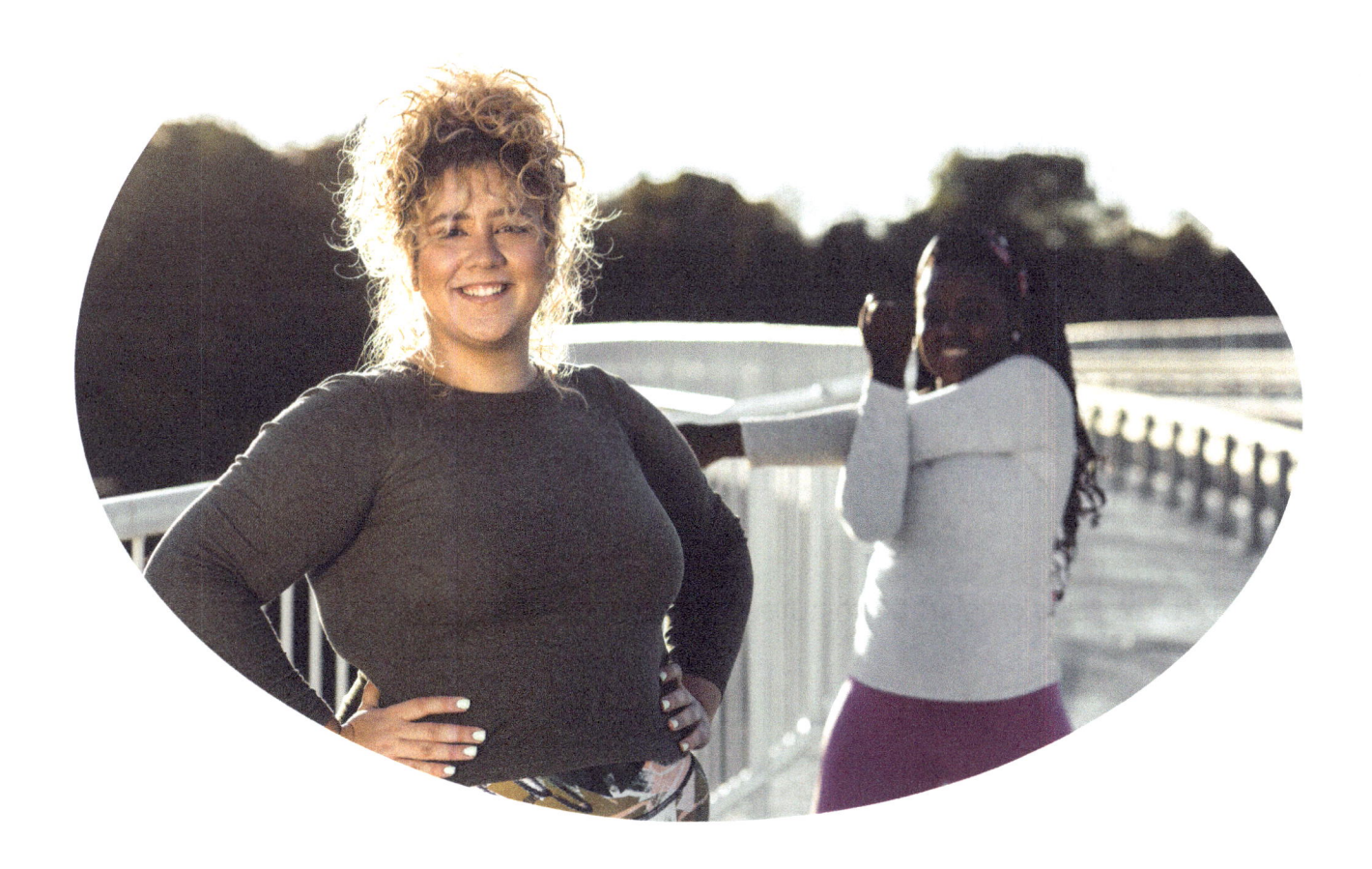

# Tips to **Keep the Weight Off**

There are no magic pills, but the habits you created while taking semaglutide can help you maintain your weight loss.

- **Eat well-balanced meals.**
  Choose meals that include protein, vegetables, fiber-rich carbohydrates and healthy fats.

- **Make protein the center of your plate.**
  Protein keeps you satisfied and helps build muscle mass. To keep the weight off, aim to eat 25-30 grams of protein per meal and if you snack, choose high-protein foods often.

- **Eat plenty of vegetables.**
  Beyond adding color and flavor to meals, vegetables can keep you satisfied for longer and add volume to your meals, helping to satisfy your hunger.

- **Add a small amount of healthy fats to your meals.**
  Fats take longer to digest, and therefore keep you fuller for longer.

- **Practice mindful eating.**
  As explained before, this practice keeps you in touch with your internal and external hunger and satiety cues.

- **Keep up physical activity.**
  Aim to exercise at least 30 minutes most days of the week.

- **Believe in yourself.**
  Research shows that self-efficacy—or believing in yourself—is associated with successful weight management.

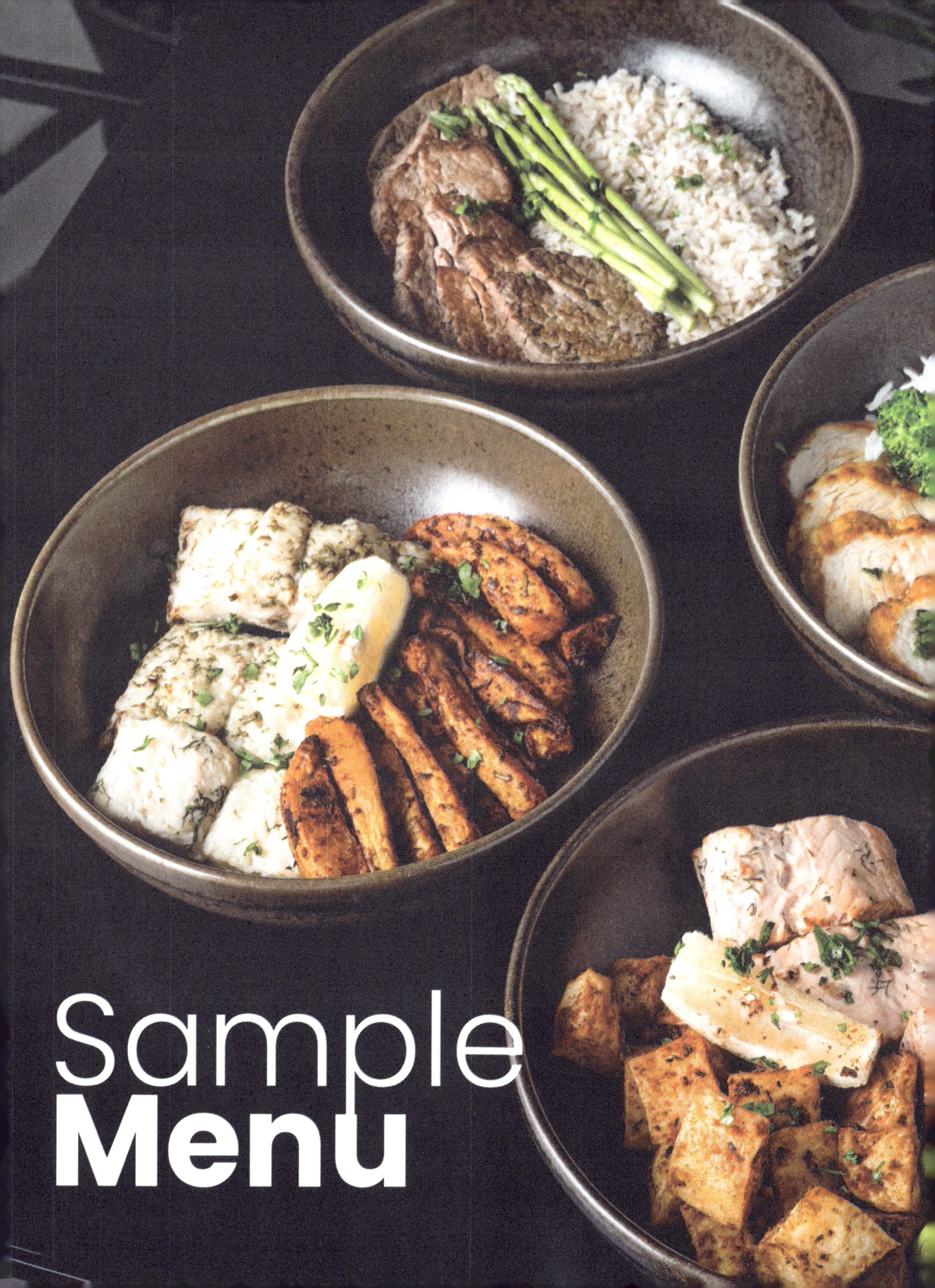

# Sample
# Menu

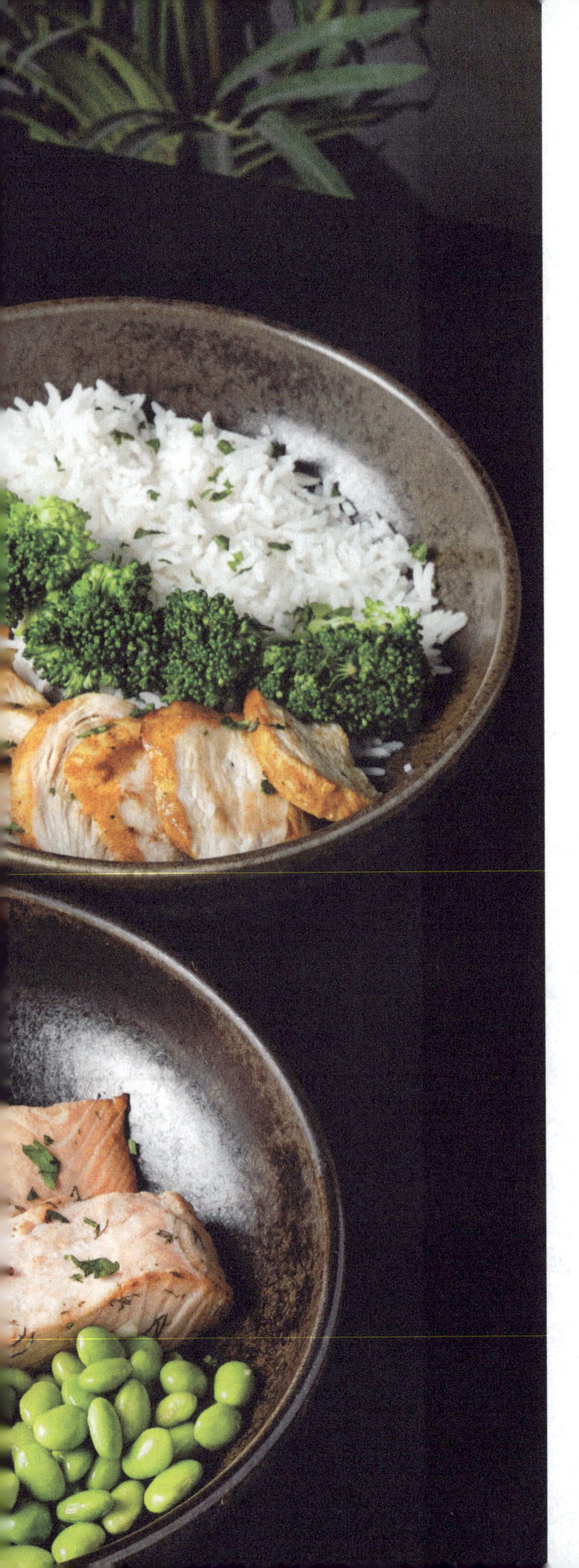

# How to use this
# sample menu

To make food planning easy for you, we have set up the sample menu so you can simply select any item from each meal list. Recipes can be found at the end of this guide.

You can make food preparation easier by doubling or tripling the recipe to make food for 2 or 3 days. Doing so can also help minimize the amount of ingredients you need to buy.

You will notice that the same ingredients are listed in several recipes. By selecting recipes with similar ingredients, you can save money at the grocery store and minimize food waste.

# Breakfast

1 protein + 1 carbohydrate + vegetables or fruit + 1 fat

Serve breakfast with coffee or tea without sugar

## Option 1
- Goat cheese and spinach omelet
- Light multigrain English muffin

## Option 2
- Avocado toast with scrambled eggs
- Fruit

## Option 3
- Overnight oats with almond butter

## Option 4
- ½ thin bagel with egg
- ½ thin bagel with almond butter and banana

## Option 5
- Chocolate oat smoothie

## Option 6
- Yogurt breakfast bowl

## Option 7
- Breakfast burrito
- Fruit

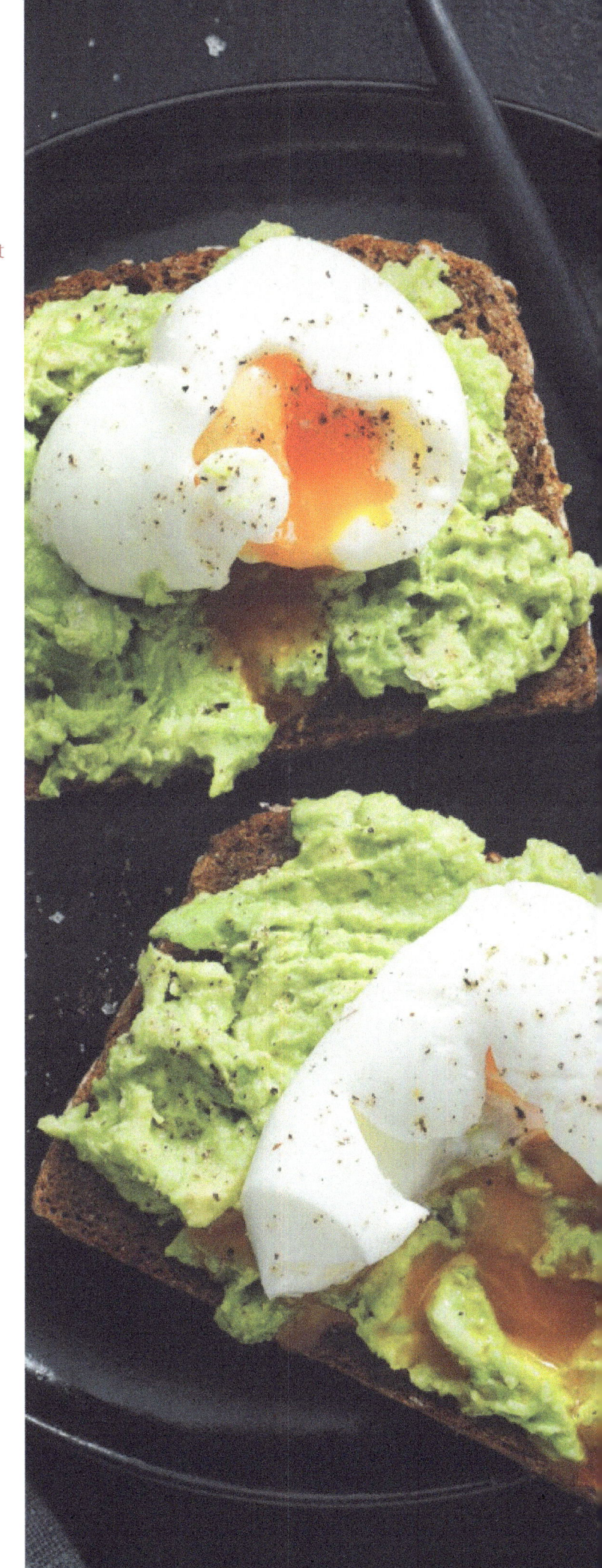

# Lunch

Pick an option here, find recipe in the next pages

1 protein + 1 carbohydrate + vegetables + 1 fat

## Option 1
- Turkey wrap

## Option 2
- Grilled chicken salad
- Thin crackers

## Option 3
- Ginger soy tofu, quinoa, and vegetable bowl (substitute the tofu for chicken, if desired)

## Option 4
- Chicken and vegetable stir fry
- Brown rice

## Option 5
- Healthy taco salad

## Option 6
- Chickpea salad

## Option 7
- Tuna salad sandwich

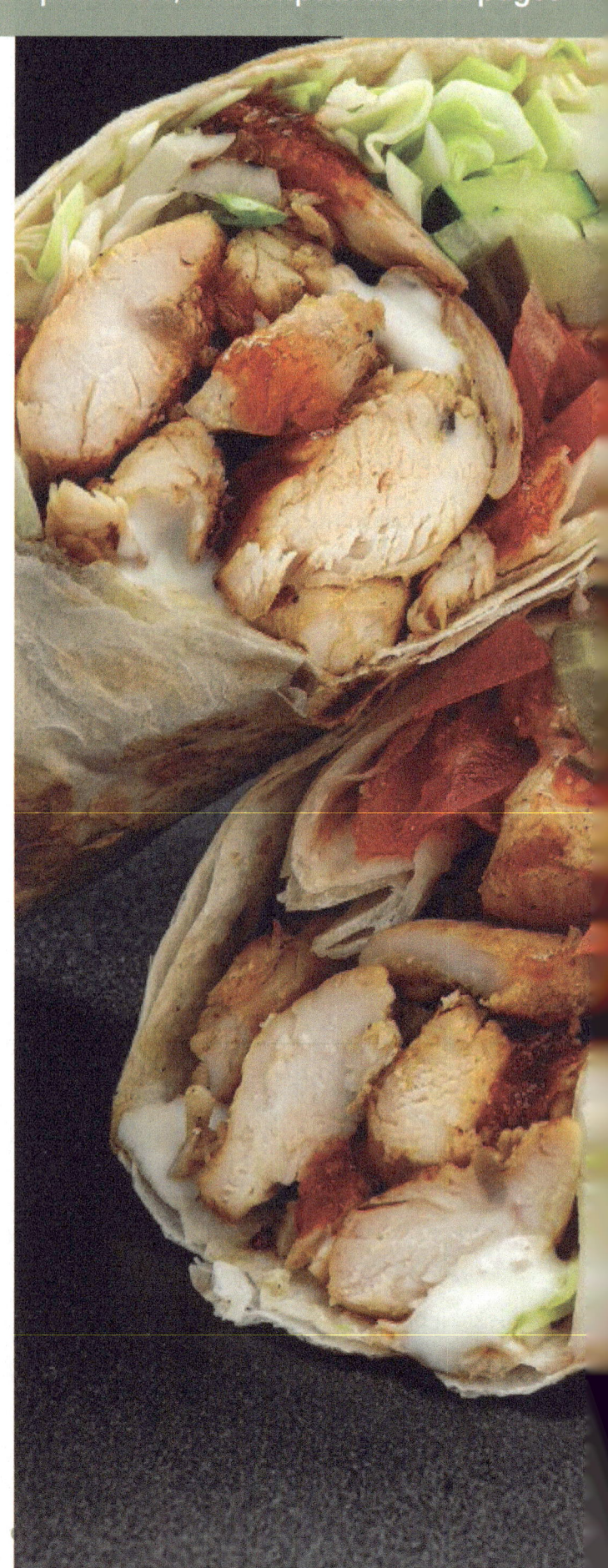

# Dinner

1 protein + vegetables + 1 fat + 1 carbohydrate (optional)

## Option 1
- Turkey meatballs with marinara sauce
- Spaghetti squash

## Option 2
- Baked salmon with tzatziki sauce
- Broccoli

## Optionb3
- Zucchini noodles with shrimp

## Option 4
- Steak salad

## Option 5
- Shrimp and vegetable stir-fry
- Cauliflower rice

## Option 6
- Mahi-mahi in papillote
- Veggies of your choice

## Option 7
- Garlic chicken, mushrooms, and cauliflower skillet

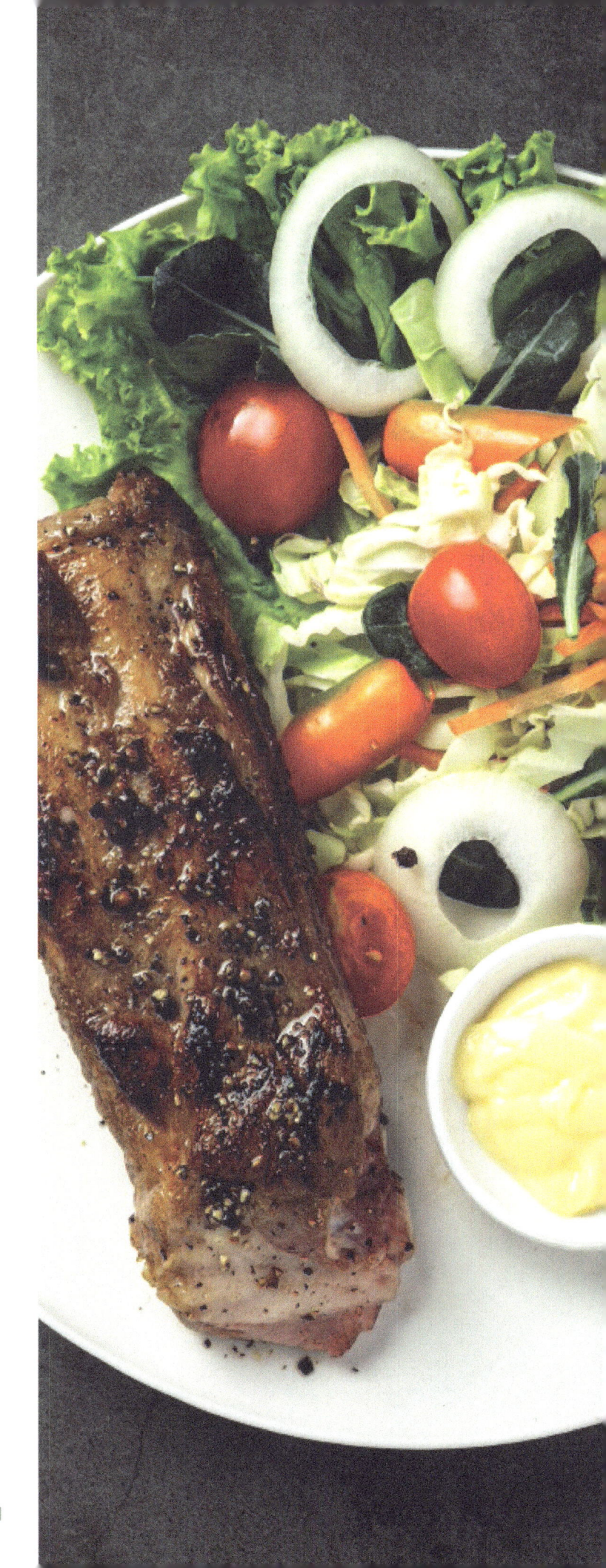

# Snack

*Pick an option here, find recipe in the next pages*

## Option 1
- Apple and 2 small pieces of dark chocolate

## Option 2
- Banana with peanut butter

## Option 3
- Protein bar

## Option 4
- Pretzels and hummus

## Option 5
- Grapes and cheese

## Option 6
- Wasa cracker
- Peanut butter

## Option 7
- Greek yogurt
- Berries

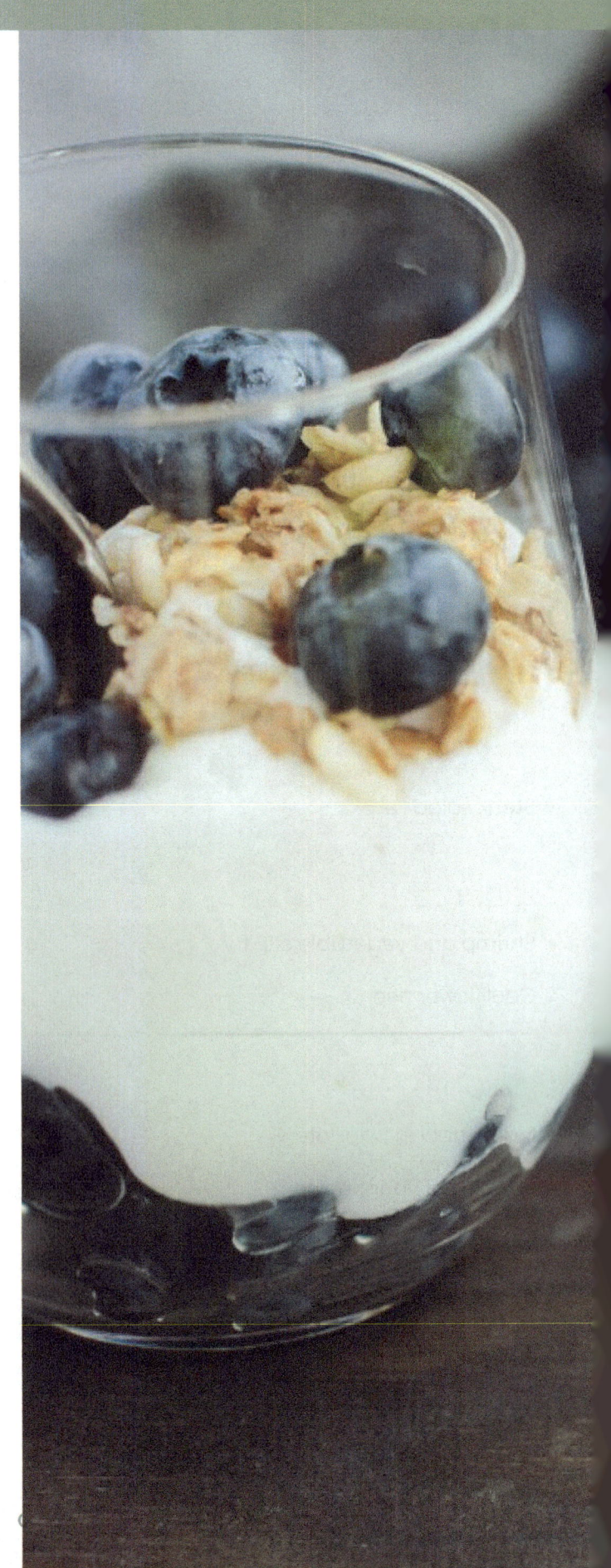

# RECIPES
## Breakfast

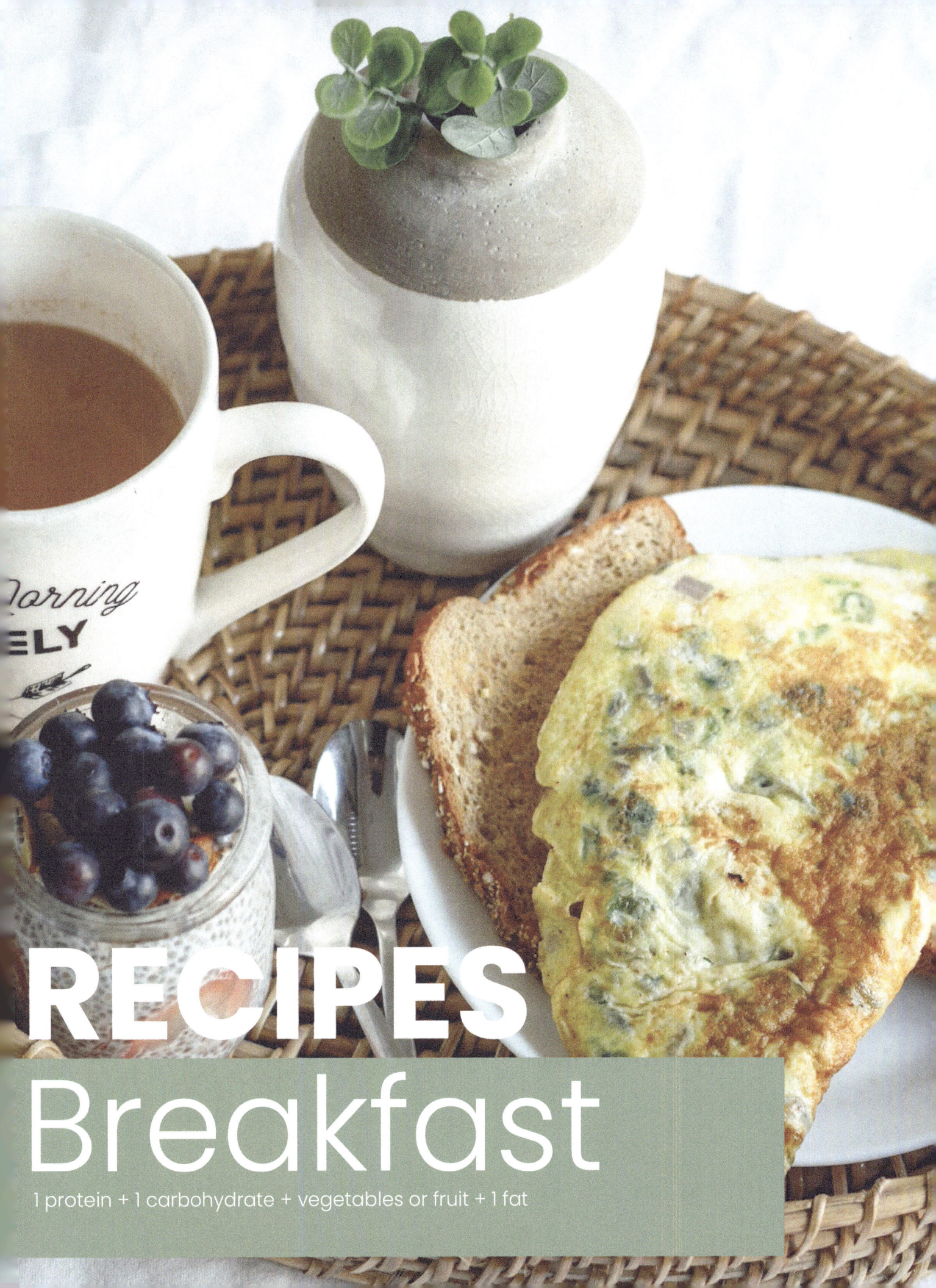

1 protein + 1 carbohydrate + vegetables or fruit + 1 fat

# Goat cheese and **spinach omelet**

## Ingredients

- Olive oil spray
- 2 eggs
- ½ cup spinach
- 1 ounce goat cheese
- 1 whole wheat English muffin

## Preparation Method

1. In a small bowl, crack the egg and beat until it's uniform in color and texture.

2. Heat a non-stick skillet over medium heat. Coat with cooking spray.

3. Add the egg mixture and cook for 1 minute without stirring until the eggs start to set.

4. Add spinach leaves and crumble goat cheese over one-half of the eggs— season with salt and pepper.

5. Gently fold the other half over the top. Cook for 30 seconds to 1 minute until the eggs are fully cooked. Use a spatula to carefully transfer to a plate.

6. Serve with a toasted English muffin.

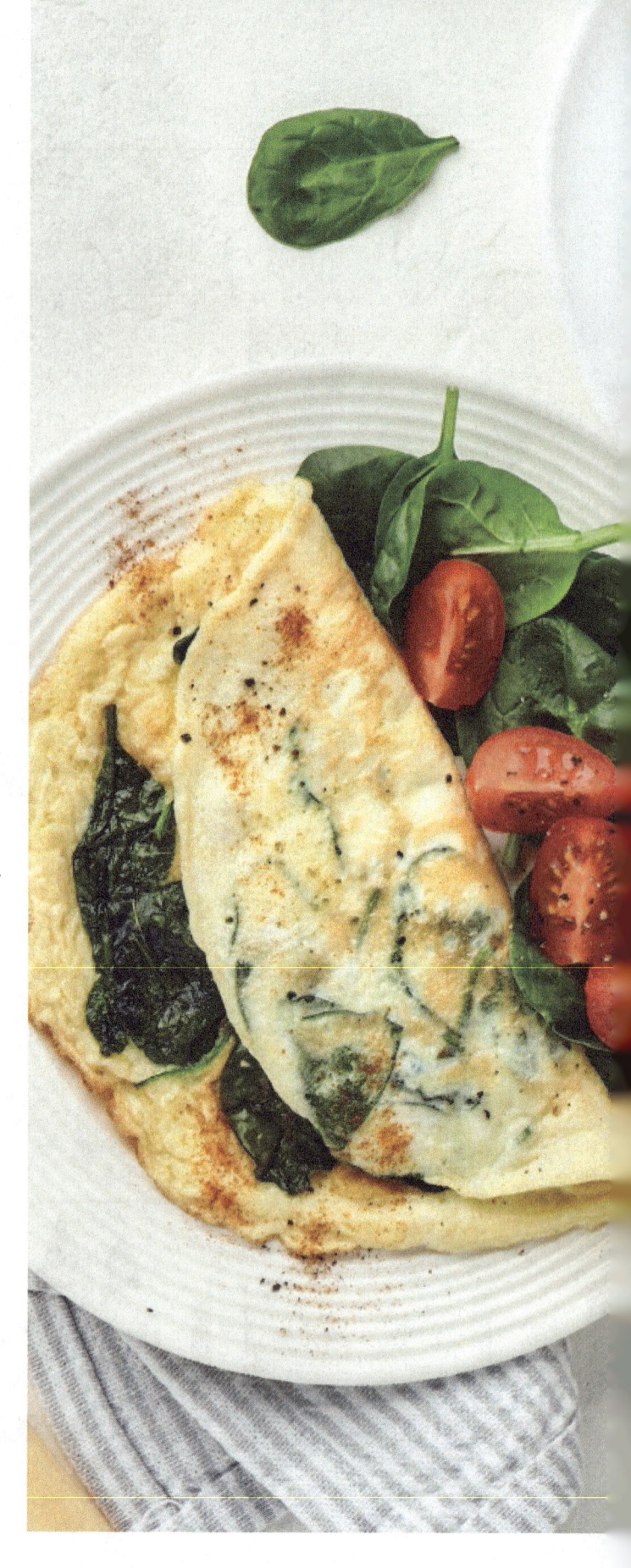

# Avocado toast with egg

### Ingredients

- 2 thin slices of sprouted bread (or bread with 3-5 g of protein per slice)
- 2 egg
- Cooking spray
- ¼ avocado
- Salt and pepper to taste
- Microgreens (optional or substitute with arugula)

### Preparation Method

1. Toast bread.

2. Slice the avocado. Arrange slices onto toast. Set aside.

3. Using cooking spray in a non-stick skillet, cook eggs using your preferred method.

4. Top your avocado toasts with the eggs.

5. Season with salt and pepper. Add the microgreens.

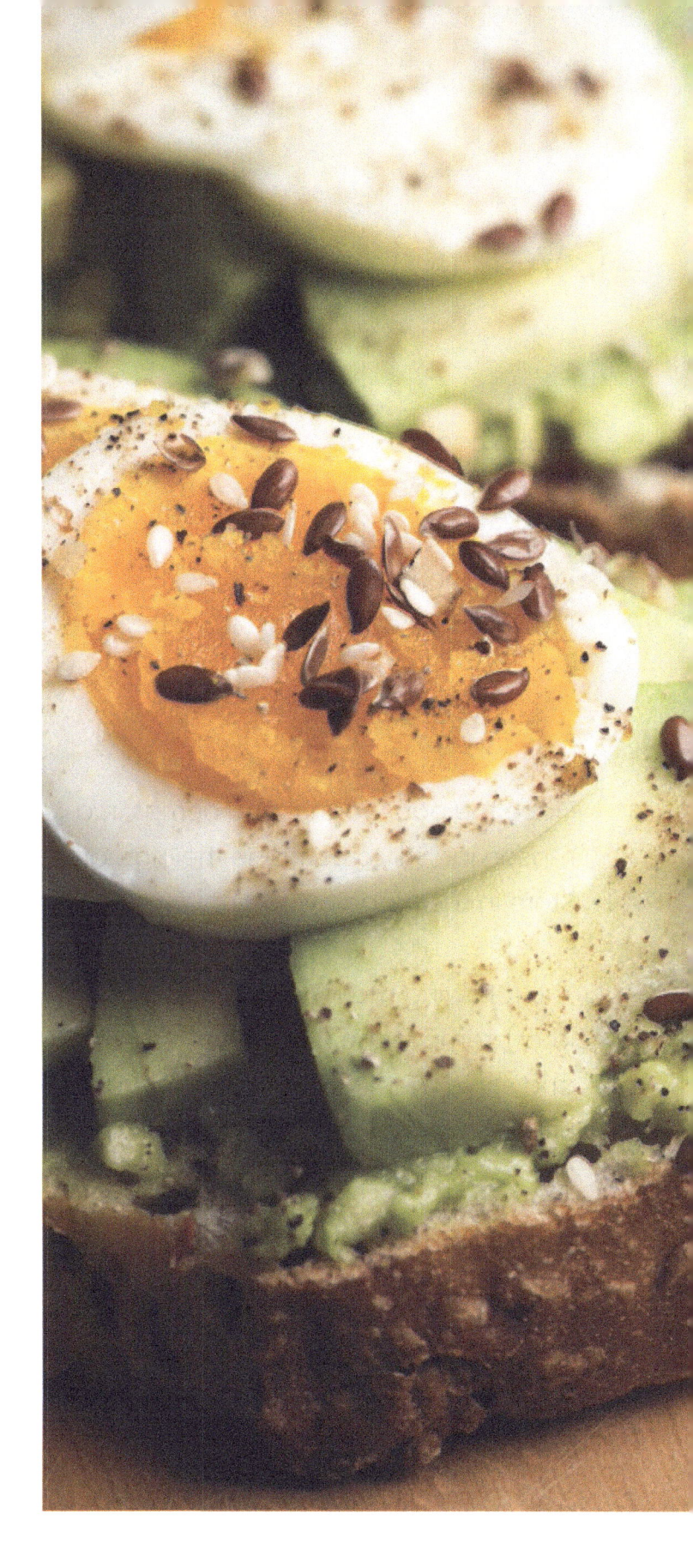

# Overnight oats

Ingredients

- ½ cup cooked oats
- ½ cup raspberries
- 1 cup plain Greek yogurt
- 1 tablespoon almond butter
- 1 teaspoon maple syrup (optional)

Preparation Method

1. Place the oats, yogurt, and berries in a mason jar. Stir to combine the ingredients. Store in the fridge overnight.

2. The following morning (or up to 5 days later), remove the mixture from the fridge and stir in maple syrup and almond butter until well combined.

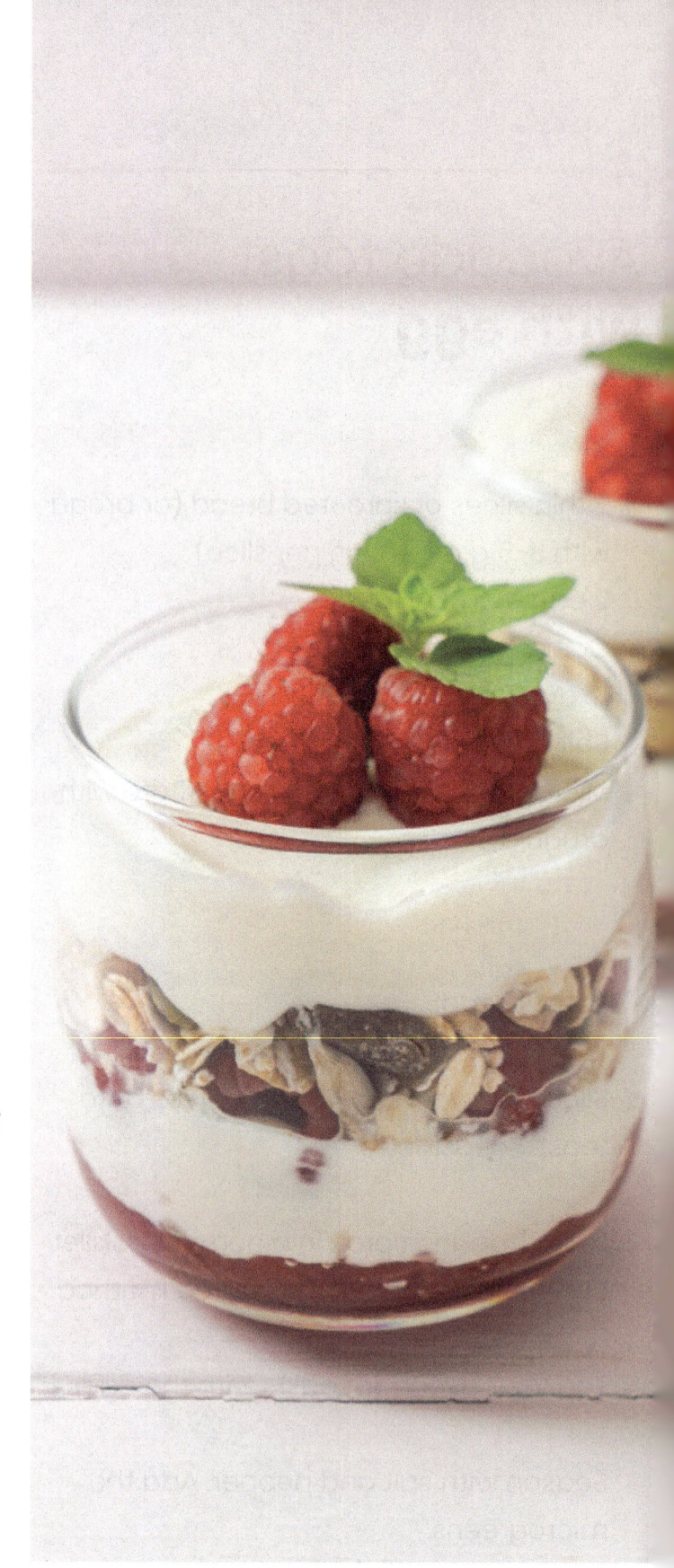

# Chocolate oat **smoothie**

## Ingredients

- ¼ cup oats
- 3 strawberries (fresh or frozen)
- ½ banana (fresh or frozen)
- 20 grams pea protein powder (chocolate flavor)
- ⅓ cup Greek yogurt (or any plant-based yogurt)
- 6 ounces unsweetened almond milk

## Preparation Method

1. Add all ingredients to a blender and mix until smooth.
2. **Enjoy!**

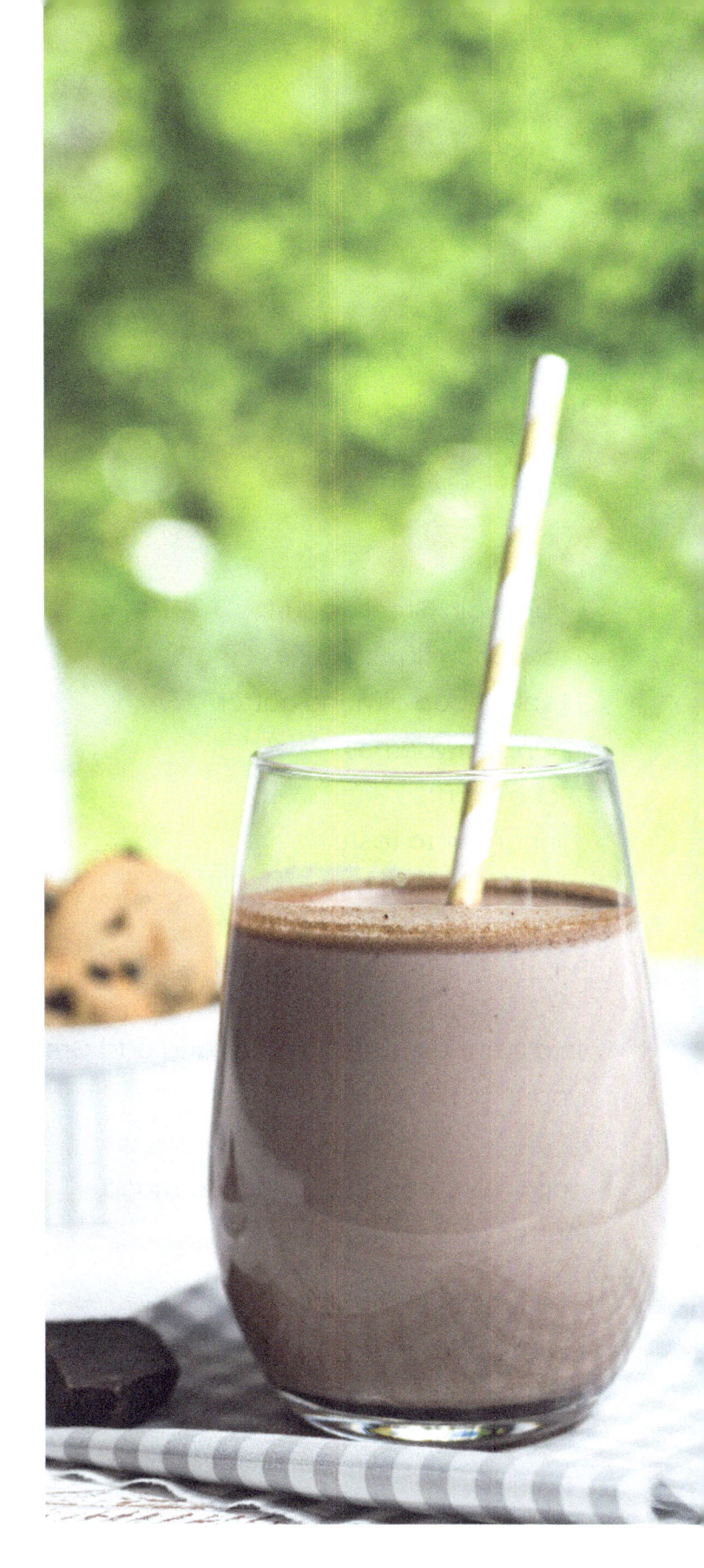

# Yogurt breakfast **bowl**

## Ingredients

- 1 cup plain Greek yogurt
- 1 teaspoon flax seeds
- 1 tablespoon almond butter
- 1 cup strawberries
- ¼ cup granola
- Cinnamon to taste

## Preparation Method

1. In a small bowl, add berries and add Greek yogurt.

2. Top with granola, flax seeds, almond butter, and cinnamon.

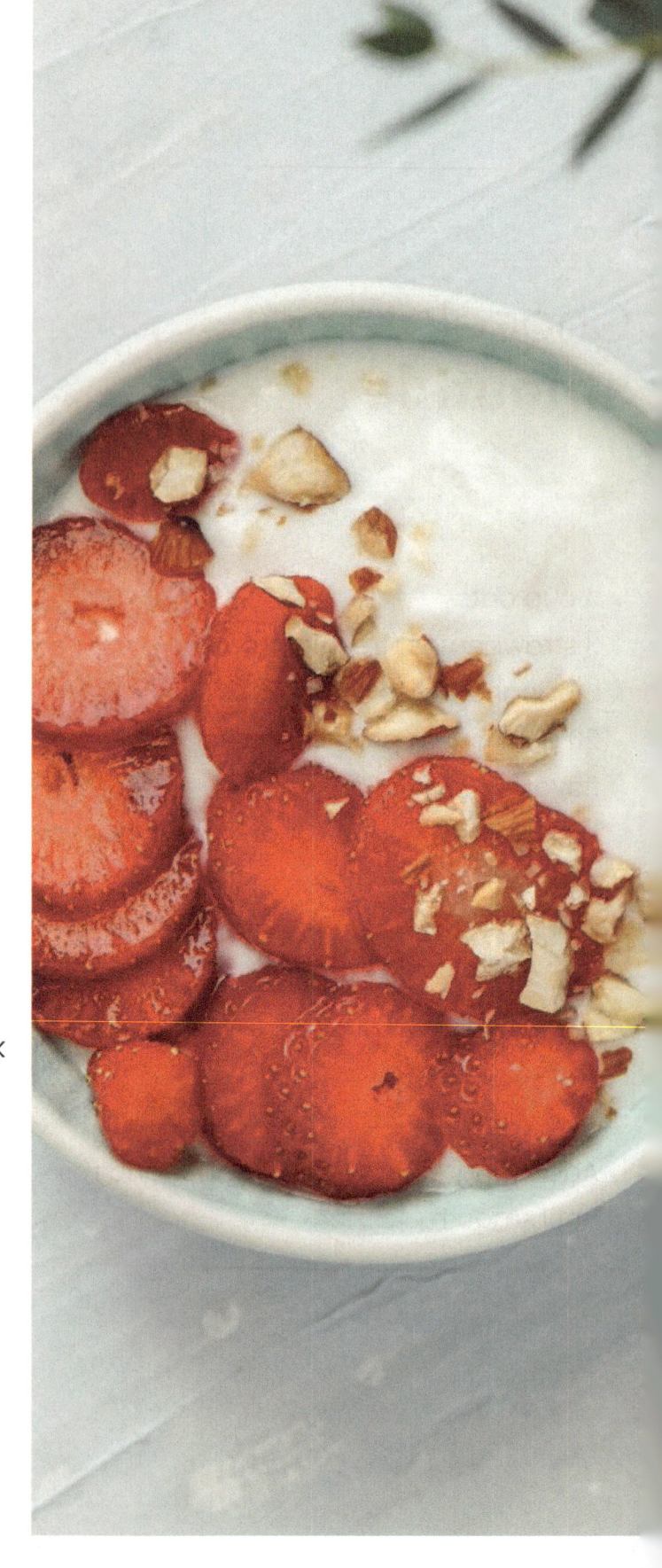

Copyright © 2024 by Dr. Su-Nui Escobar, RDN, LDN

# Breakfast
# **burrito**

## Ingredients

- Cooking spray
- 2 eggs
- ¼ avocado, sliced
- 1 low-carb wrap
- Salt and pepper to taste
- Salsa (optional)

## Preparation Method

1. In a small bowl, beat eggs. Set aside.

2. Spray a non-stick pan with cooking spray. Add the egg mixture and cook to your desired consistency. Remove from heat.

3. While the egg is cooking, warm the tortilla in a skillet.

4. Place the tortilla on a plate, and add sliced avocado and eggs. Top with salsa, roll, and enjoy. You could fold in the ends of the tortilla, but in Mexico, we just roll burritos!

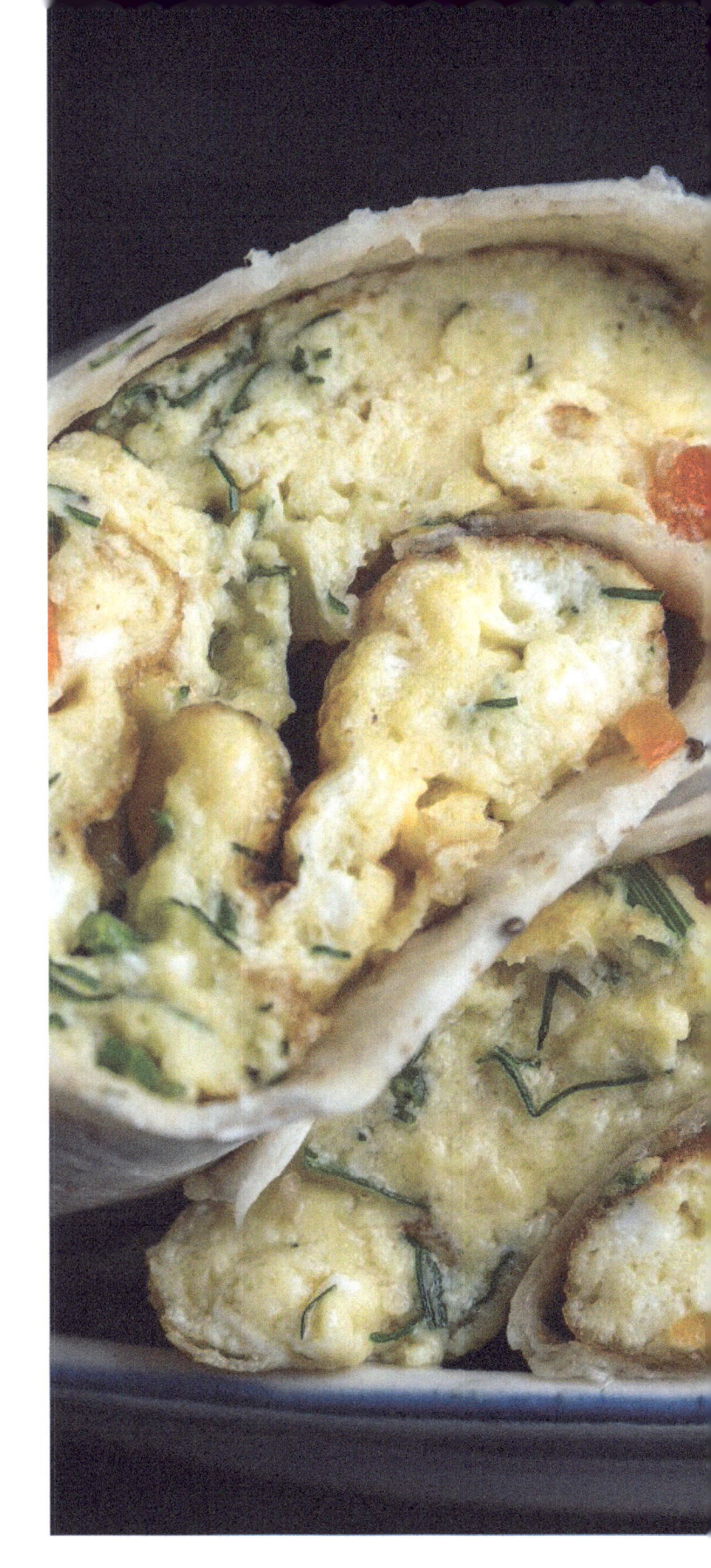

# Lunch

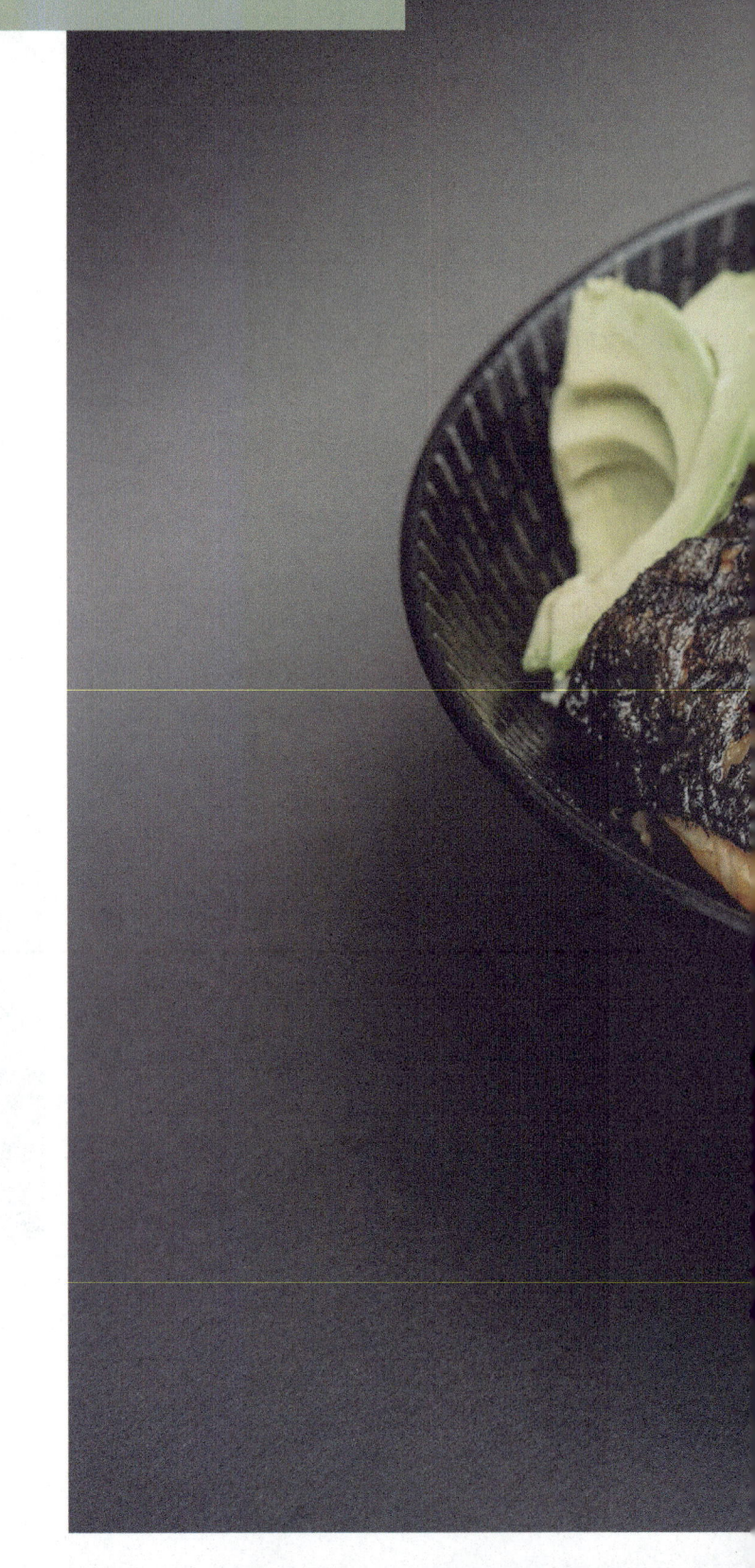

# Turkey **wrap**

### Ingredients

- 1 low-carb wrap
- 1 slice cheese
- 3 ounces of sliced turkey
- Shredded lettuce or spinach and tomato

### Preparation Method

1. On a large plate, lay the wrap flat.

2. Layer the turkey, cheese, lettuce, and tomato slices over the wrap.

3. Roll wrap while simultaneously tucking the ends.

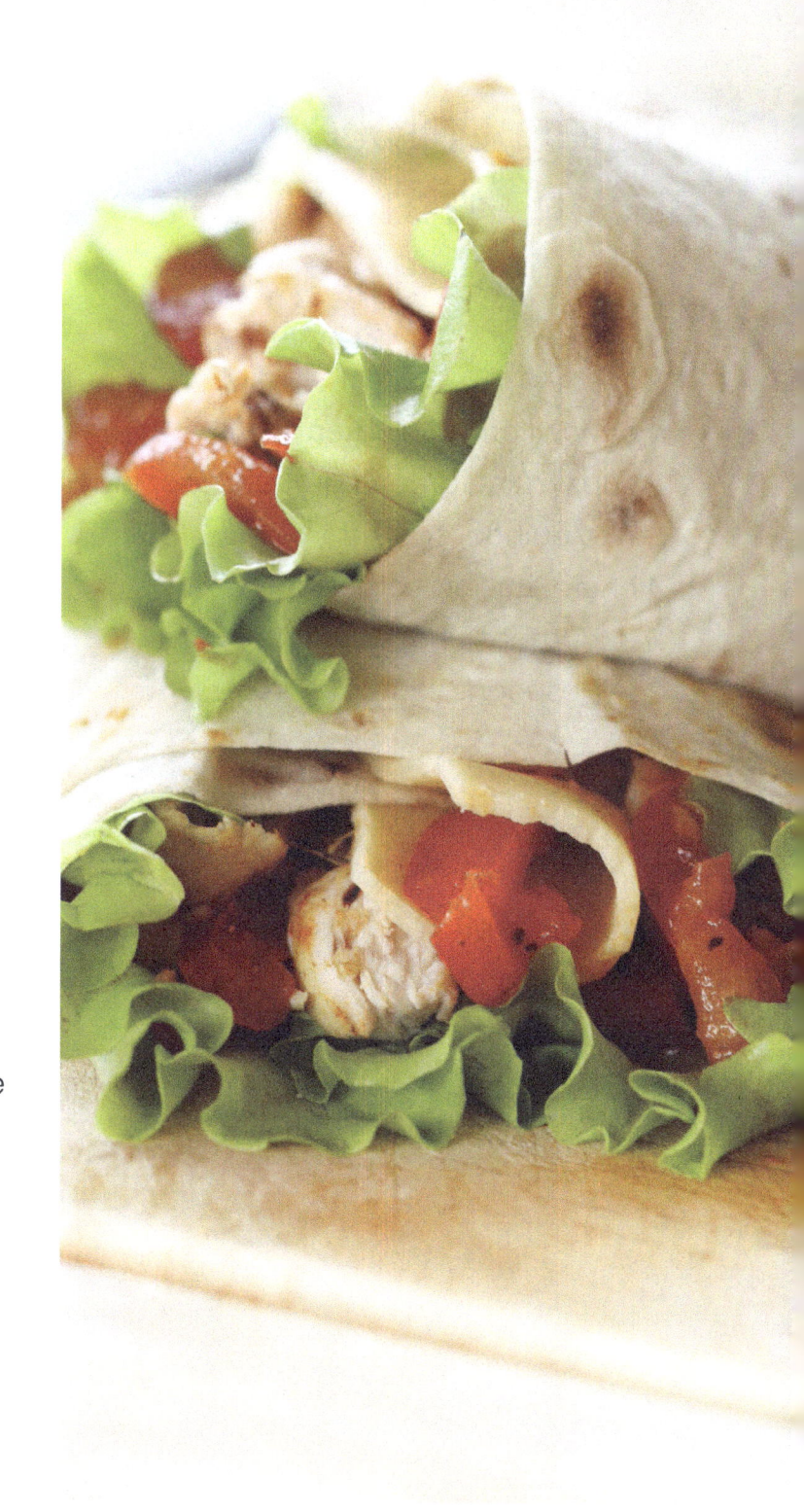

Copyright © 2024 by Dr. Su-Nui Escobar, RDN, LDN

# Grilled chicken **salad with quinoa**

### Ingredients

- 4 ounces grilled chicken
- 2 cups mixed greens, arugula, or spinach
- ½ cup quinoa, cooked
- 4 cherry tomatoes, halved
- ½ cucumber, chopped
- 2 tablespoons light vinaigrette

### Preparation Method

1. In a medium bowl, combine all vegetables. Add vinaigrette and toss. Top with quinoa and chicken.

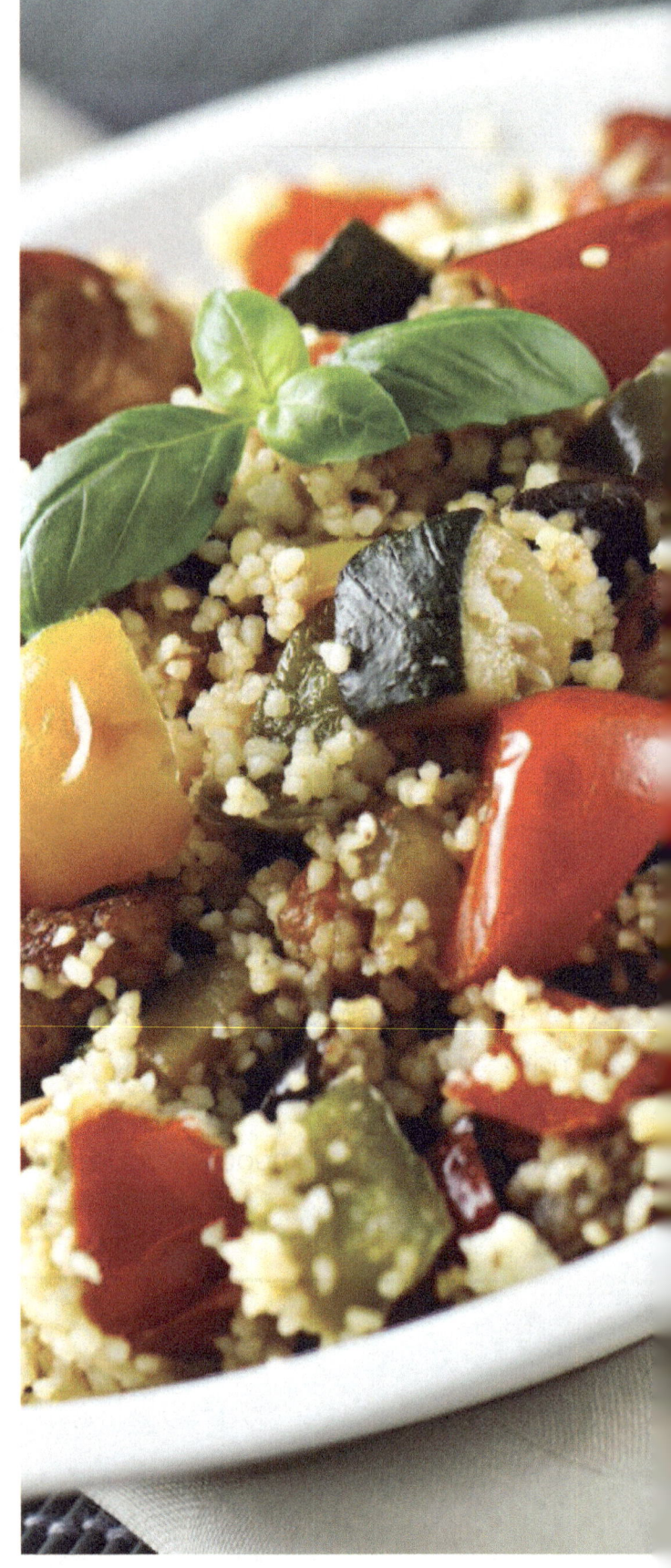

# Ginger soy tofu, brown rice, and vegetable bowl

## Ingredients
### Tofu

- 6 ounces extra firm tofu (substitute chicken for tofu, if desired)
- 1 teaspoon soy sauce or liquid aminos
- 1 teaspoon cornstarch
- 1 tablespoon fresh ginger, grated (or ½ tablespoon ground)
- 1 garlic clove, minced
- 1 tablespoon rice vinegar
- 1 tablespoon olive oil
- Cooking spray

### For the bowl

- ½ cup quinoa
- ⅓ cup shredded purple cabbage
- ⅓ cup shredded carrots
- ⅓ cup sliced cucumber
- ⅓ cup shelled edamame
- 2 slices avocado

## Preparation Method

1. Drain the block of tofu and wrap it in a clean kitchen towel. Press with a plate or book for a few minutes to remove extra liquid while you prepare the marinade.

2. Cook quinoa according to package instructions.

3. In a small bowl, mix soy sauce, cornstarch, ginger, garlic, and rice vinegar.

4. Cut tofu into cubes and add to marinade. Let it rest for 5-10 minutes.

5. In a small skillet, add olive oil and tofu. Cook until brown. Remove tofu from the skillet and set aside.

6. In a bowl, add quinoa, tofu, vegetables and avocado.

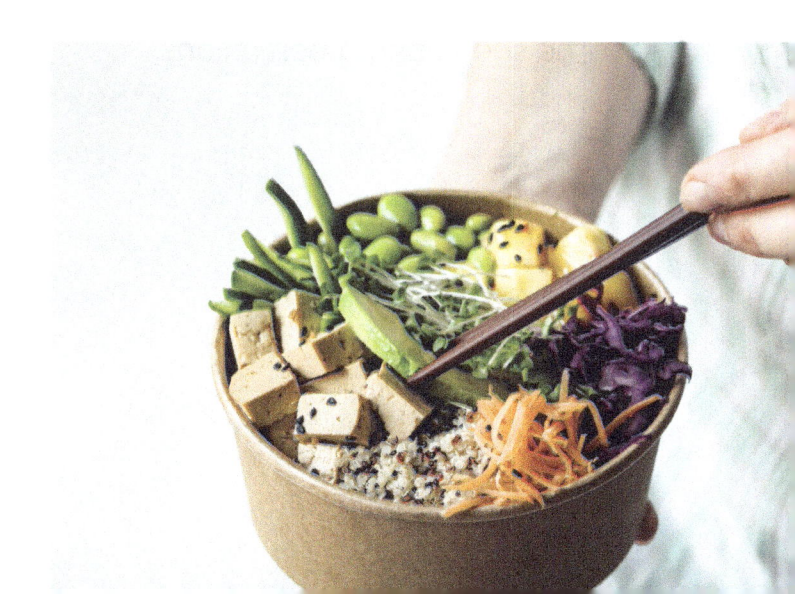

# Chicken **stir-fry**

Ingredients

- 4 ounces chicken
- Cooking spray
- 1 cup brown rice, cooked
- 1 cup broccoli, chopped
- 1 tablespoon green onions, sliced
- ½ Tbsp sesame seeds, toasted
- 1 tablespoon soy sauce

Preparation Method

1. Cut chicken into slices.

2. Spray a medium non-stick skillet with cooking spray. Add chicken and cook, over medium heat, until brown from both sides. Add soy sauce

3. Add vegetables and cook for 4-5 minutes until tender. Serve over rice and top with sesame seeds and green onions.

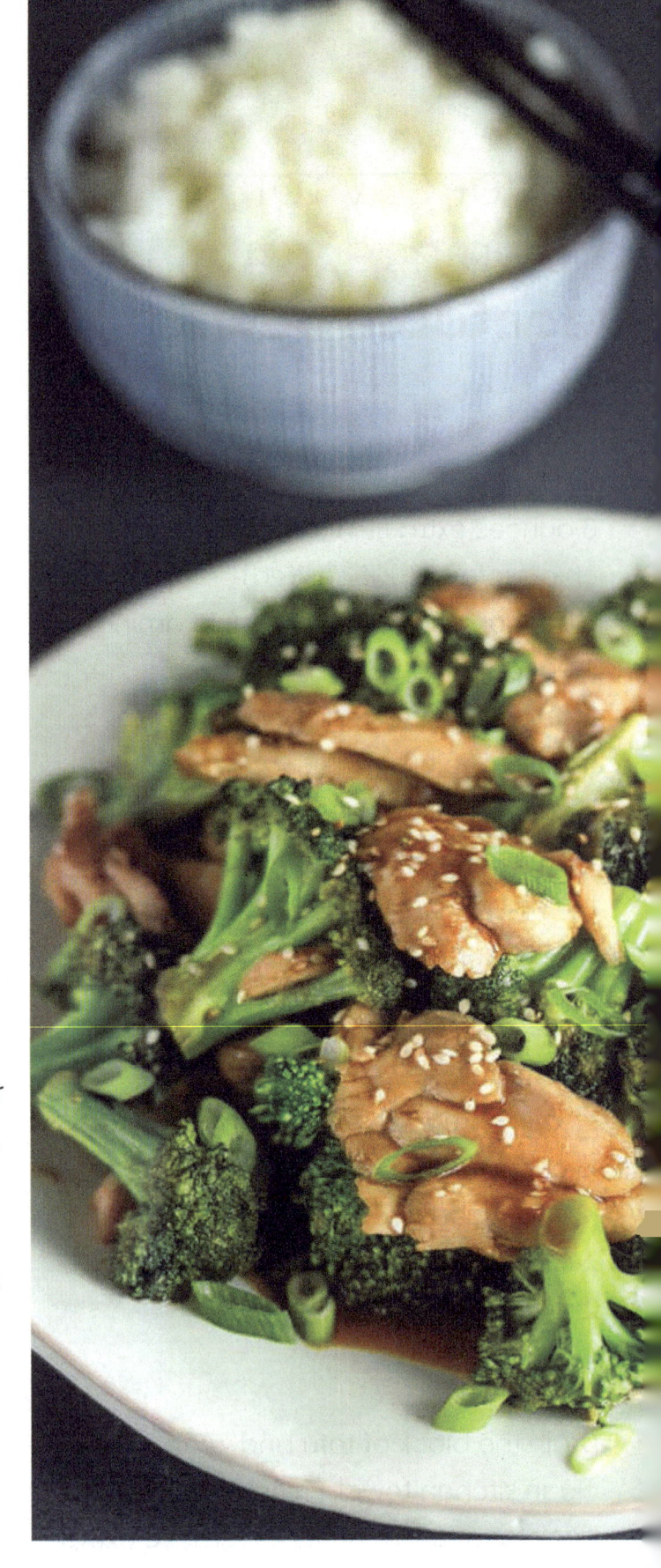

Copyright © 2024 by Dr. Su-Nui Escobar, RDN, LDN

# Healthy taco **salad**

### Ingredients

- Cooking spray
- 4 ounces lean ground bison (or lean
- ground beef)
- Salt and pepper
- ½ tablespoon taco seasoning to taste
- 1 tablespoon water
- 1 cup beans, cooked
- 2 tablespoons romaine lettuce
- 4 cherry tomatoes, halved
- ⅓ hass avocado
- 2 tablespoons salsa
- 1 tablespoon sour cream

### Preparation Method

1. Place a nonstick skillet over medium heat and add cooking spray. Add ground bison. Cook for 2 minutes.

2. Break apart the meat and flip it over. Cook until brown. Season with salt and pepper.

3. Add taco seasoning and water. Reduce the heat to low and let it simmer, stirring occasionally.

4. Cook for about 1-2 minutes until the liquid is mostly gone. Add beans and cook for another 2 minutes.

5. In a serving bowl, add lettuce, tomatoes, and avocado.

6. Place the cooked seasoned beef on top, followed by salsa and sour cream.

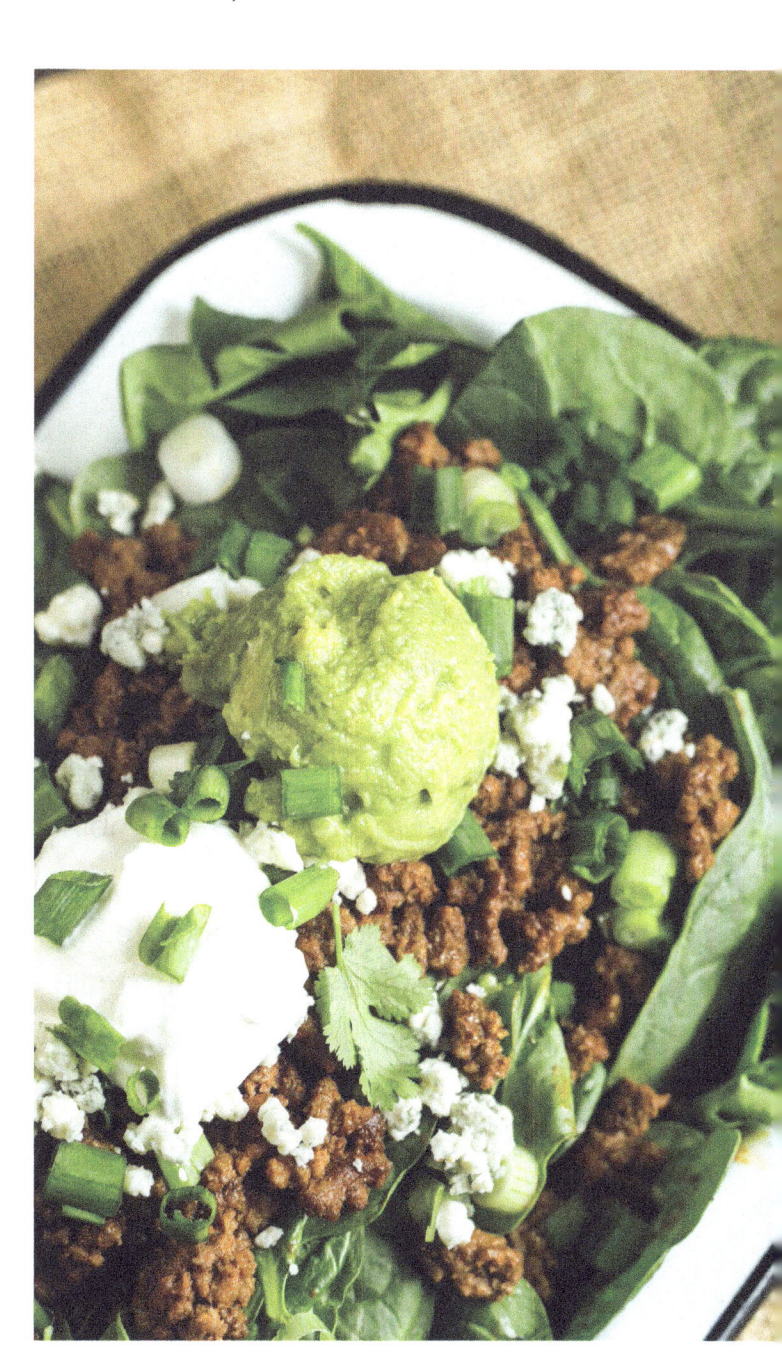

# Chickpea salad

### Ingredients

- 1 cup chickpeas
- ½ cucumber, diced
- 1 medium roma tomato, diced
- ½ small shallot, chopped
- 1-ounce reduced-fat feta, crumbled
- 1 tablespoon parsley
- 1 lemon
- Salt and pepper to taste

### Preparation Method

1. Combine chickpeas, cucumber, tomato, shallot, reduced-fat feta cheese, and parsley in a medium mixing bowl.

2. Add the lemon juice and season with salt and black pepper to taste. Stir to combine.

3. The salad can be enjoyed immediately but is best served chilled. Cover and chill in the fridge for at least 1 hour.

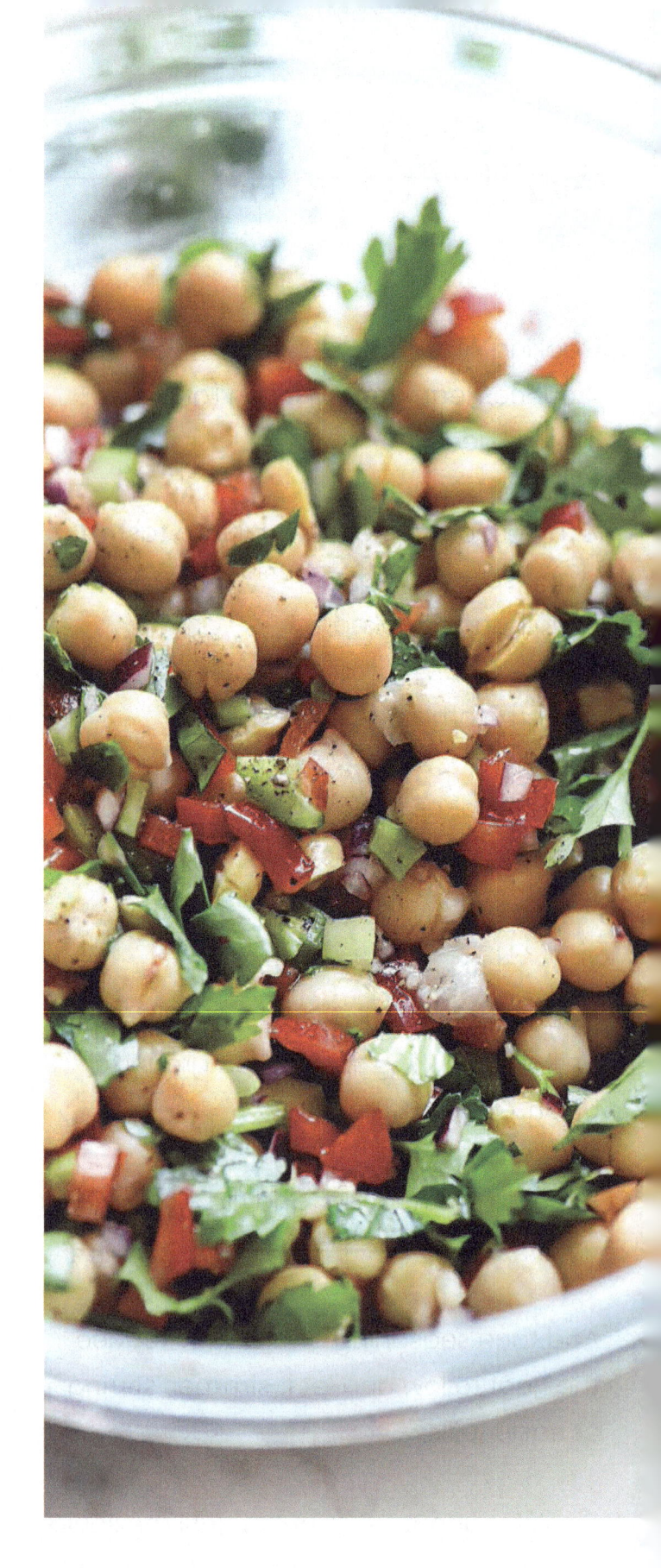

# Tuna salad **sandwich**

## Ingredients

- 3 ounces canned tuna packed in water
- ½ cup nonfat plain Greek yogurt
- ¼ cup diced celery
- 1 tablespoon Dijon mustard
- ¼ teaspoon salt, to taste
- ¼ teaspoon pepper, to taste
- 2 slices whole wheat bread

## Preparation Method

1. In a bowl, combine tuna, Greek yogurt, celery, mustard, salt, and pepper. Mix well.

2. Toast the slices of bread (optional).

3. Assemble the sandwich.

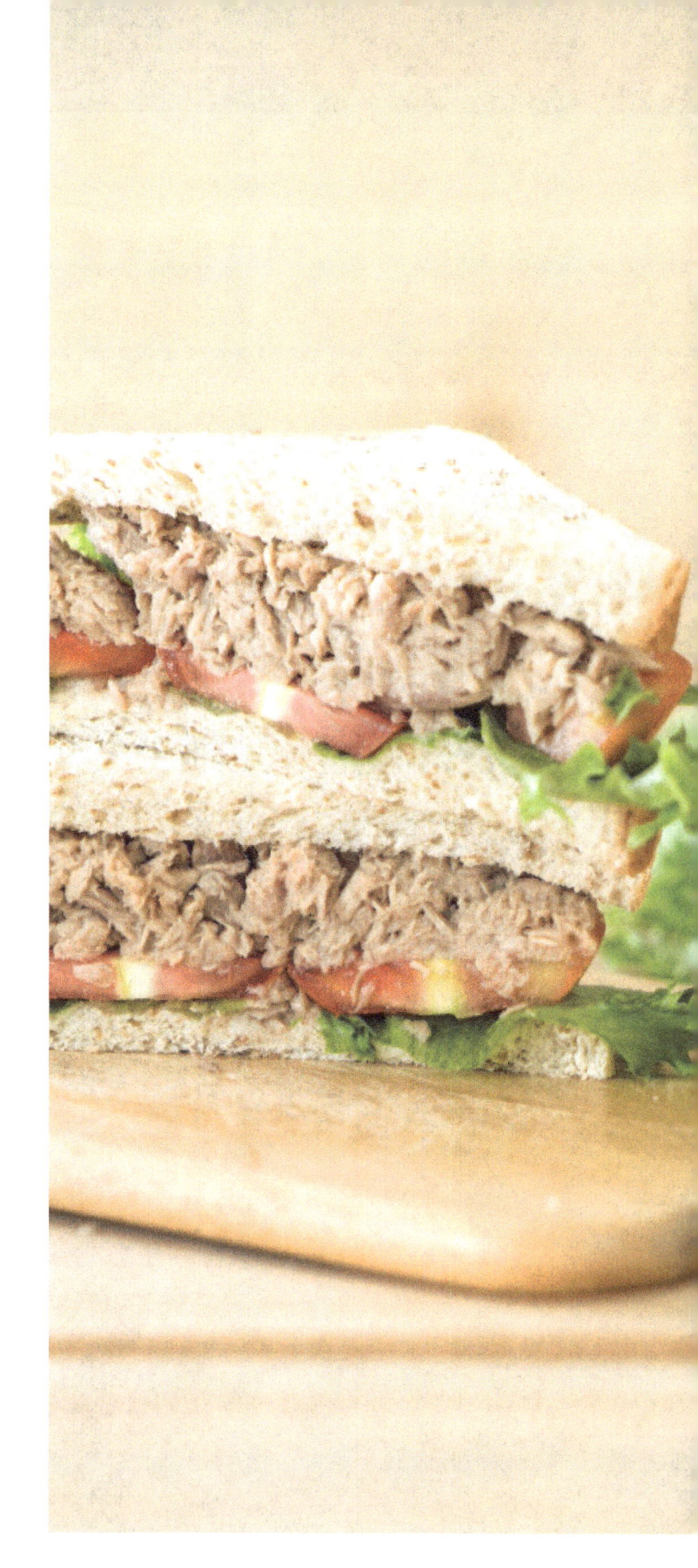

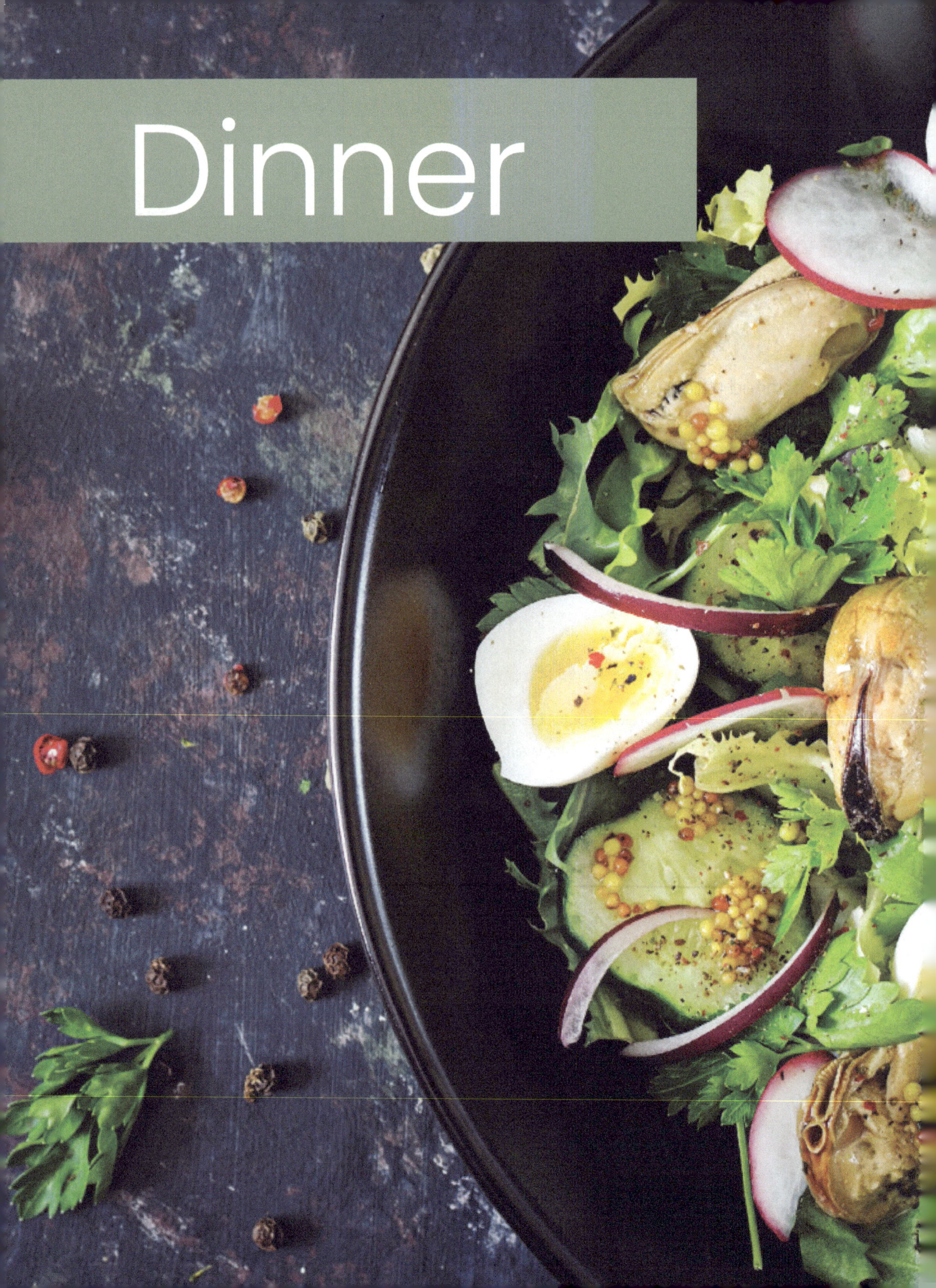

# Dinner

# Turkey meatballs
# with marinara sauce

## Ingredients

- 4 ounces ground turkey
- 1 tablespoon panko
- 1 tablespoon parmesan cheese, grated
- ½ egg
- Salt and pepper to taste
- ½ cup marinara sauce
- Zucchini noodles (or another low-carb pasta alternative)
- Additional grated parmesan cheese

## Preparation Method

1. Preheat oven to 400°F. Line a baking sheet with parchment paper.

2. In a bowl, combine ground turkey, panko, egg, grated cheese, salt, and pepper.

3. Using your hands, form the mixture into individual 1-inch balls.

4. Place meatballs on the baking sheet and bake for 20 minutes.

5. In a non-stick skillet, add cooking spray and cook zucchini noodles. Add marinara sauce and mix.

6. Serve in a serving bowl and add meatballs. Top with cheese.

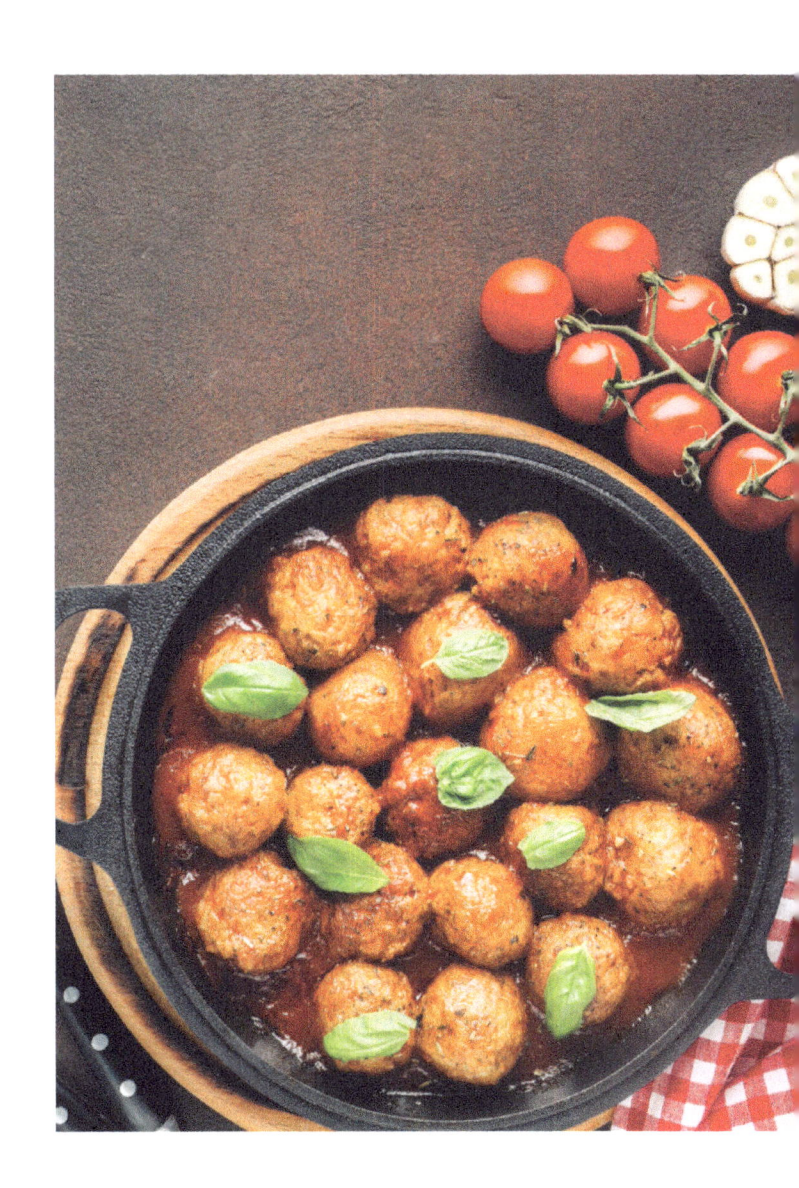

Copyright © 2024 by Dr. Su-Nui Escobar, RDN, LDN

# Baked salmon
## with tzatziki sauce

### Ingredients
**Salmon**

- 4 ounces salmon
- 1 lime or lemon, juiced
- ½ teaspoon dill, fresh or dried
- Salt and pepper to taste
- 1 cup broccoli florets

**Tzatziki sauce**

- ½ cup non-fat Greek yogurt
- ¼ cup cucumber, finely chopped
- ½ tablespoon dill, chopped
- ½ tablespoon lemon juice
- Sprig of mint, chopped (optional)
- Salt and pepper to taste

### Preparation Method

1. Preheat oven to 400°F.

2. Line a baking sheet with parchment paper. Place salmon on parchment paper and season with the juice of the lime or lemon, salt and pepper, and dill. Place broccoli florets on the side and season with salt and pepper.

3. Bake for 20-25 minutes or until fully cooked.

4. Prepare the sauce: In a medium bowl, combine the cucumber, yogurt, lemon juice, olive oil, garlic, salt, dill, and mint, if using. Chill until ready to use.

5. Serve salmon with tzatziki sauce on top.

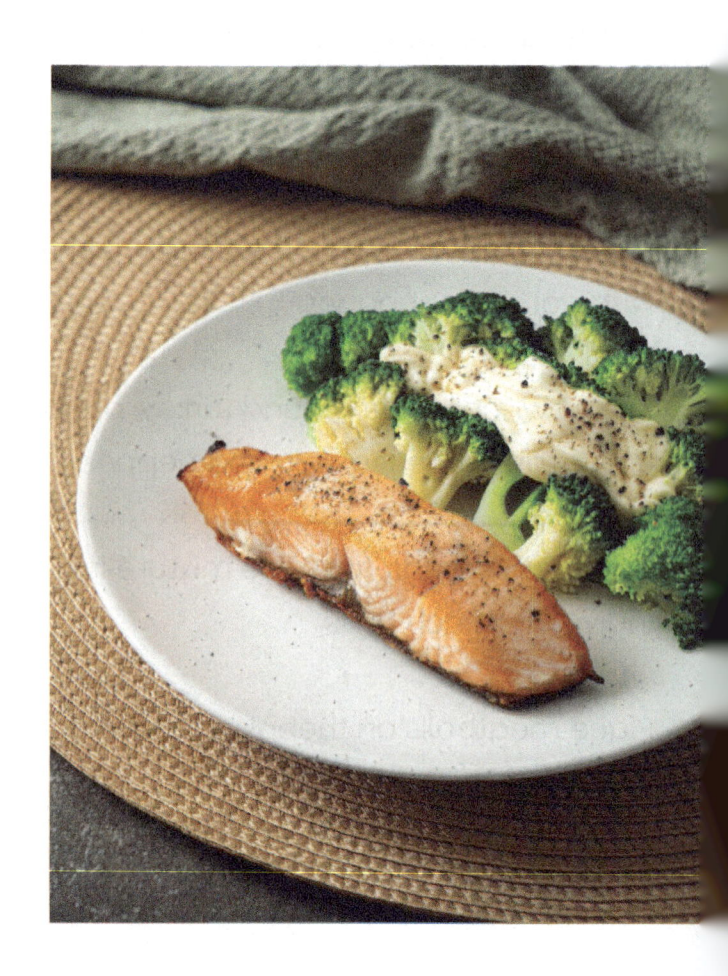

# Zucchini noodles with shrimp

## Ingredients

- 1 tablespoon olive oil
- ¼ onion, chopped
- 1 garlic cloves
- 5 ounces shrimp
- Salt and pepper to taste
- Red chili flakes
- ½ cup chicken broth
- ½ teaspoon dill (more for garnish)
- 1 lemon
- 1 cup zucchini noodles

## Preparation Method

1. Add olive oil to a non-stick skillet. Place over medium heat. Add the onions and cook until beginning to soften, about 2 minutes.

2. Add the garlic and cook for 30 seconds. Add the shrimp, salt, pepper, and red pepper flakes. Cook the shrimp in a sauté for 3 minutes until they start to cook but are still somewhat see-through.

3. Add the chicken broth, dill, and lemon juice. To cook the shrimp, bring them to a boil and let them cook for 1 minute until fully opaque.

4. Add the zucchini noodles and toss with the shrimp so that they are coated with the garlic lemon sauce. Do not overcook the zucchini noodles to keep the consistency.

5. Plate the dish. Sprinkle with dill. Serve warm.

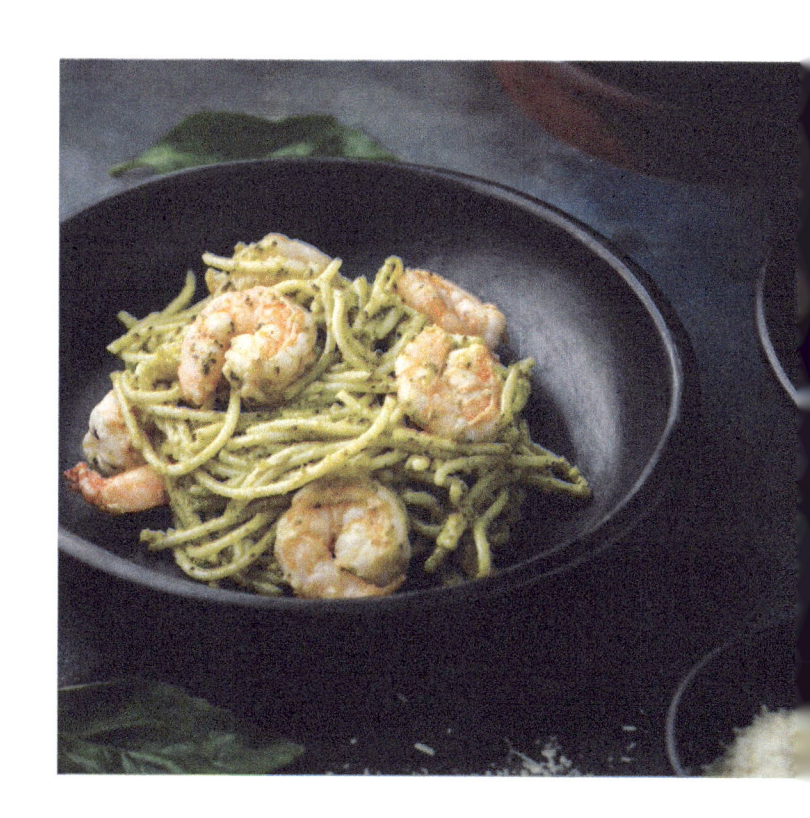

Copyright © 2024 by Dr. Su-Nui Escobar, RDN, LDN

# Steak **salad**

## Ingredients

- Cooking spray
- 4 ounces steak, sliced
- 1 cup green or red bell peppers, sliced
- 1 cup red onions, sliced
- 2 cups arugula or romaine lettuce
- 4 cherry tomatoes, halved
- 1 ounce feta cheese
- 2 tablespoons pico de gallo

## Preparation Method

1. In a non-stick skillet, add cooking spray. Sautee onions and peppers until soft. Remove from heat and set aside.

2. In the same skillet, add more cooking spray and the steak. Cook for 3 minutes on one side. Turn and cook an additional 3 minutes. Cook longer for a well cooked steak. Remove from heat and set aside.

3. Combine the arugula or lettuce, cherry tomatoes, and cheese in a bowl. Toss the salad with vinaigrette. Season the salad with salt and pepper to taste and transfer to a plate.

4. Arrange the steak slices on top of the salad and top with sauteed onions and peppers. Add pico de gallo.

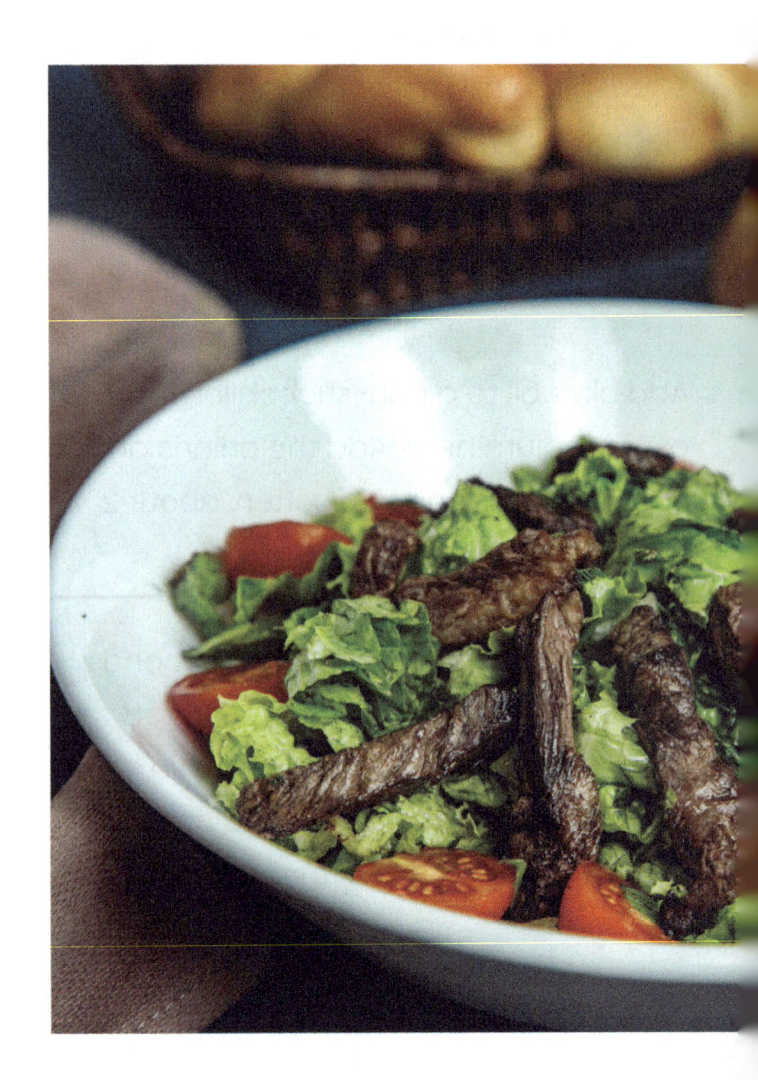

# Mahi-mahi en papillote

## Ingredients

- 4 ounces mahi-mahi
- 2 tablespoon cooking wine
- 1 teaspoon fresh or ½ teaspoon dried dill
- Salt and pepper to taste
- ½ cup carrot cut lengthwise
- ½ cup zucchini, cut lengthwise
- 1 tablespoon slivered almonds
- 1 tablespoon butter
- 1 package ready-made cauliflower rice

## Preparation Method

1. Preheat oven to 375°F.
2. Place each mahi-mahi fillet portion on a piece of parchment or heavy-duty foil.
3. Drizzle fish with wine. Add dill, salt, and pepper. Then add carrot, zucchini, almonds, and butter.
4. Wrap the fish in foil or parchment, ensuring it is tightly sealed. Place packets on a baking sheet.
5. Bake until the fish flakes easily with a fork, 15-20 minutes. Carefully open the foil to let out the steam.
6. Make cauliflower rice according to package instructions.
7. Serve the fish with rice.

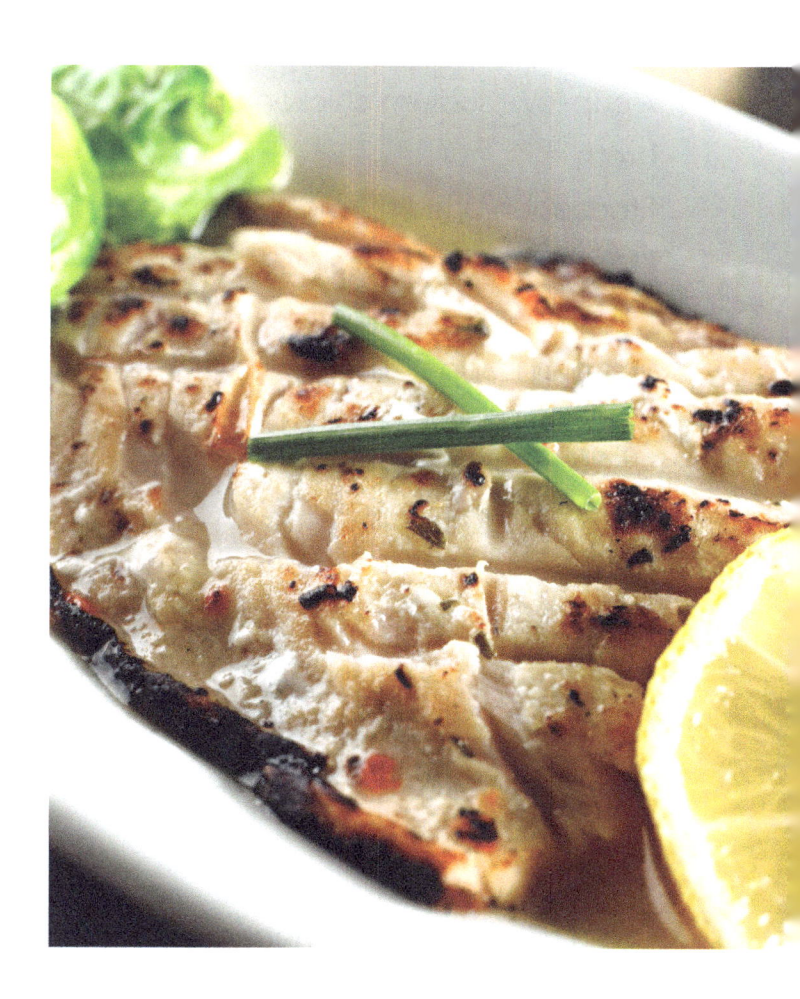

# Garlic mushrooms, chicken, **and** cauliflower skillet

### Ingredients

Cooking spray
4 ounces chicken breast, sliced
1 tablespoon olive oil
¼ onion, chopped
¼ head cauliflower, cut into florets
1 cup mushrooms, washed and cleaned
¼ cup low-sodium chicken or vegetable broth
1 teaspoon dried thyme
1 teaspoon dried parsley
1 garlic clove, minced
Salt and pepper to taste

### Preparation Method

1. Heat a non-stick skillet and add cooking spray. Add chicken and cook for 3-4 minutes, turn and cook for additional 3-4 minutes or until chicken is cooked through. Remove the chicken from the skillet and set aside.

2. Using the same skillet, heat oil over medium-high heat. Sauté the onion until softened, approximately 3 minutes.

3. Add the mushrooms and cook for about 4-5 minutes. Remove any liquid.

4. Add cauliflower florets. Cook until golden and crispy on the edges, about 8-10 minutes.

5. Add chicken and garlic.

6. Pour in the broth, stir, and cook for 2 minutes.

7. Add thyme and parsley. Cook for an additional minute. Season with salt and pepper to taste.

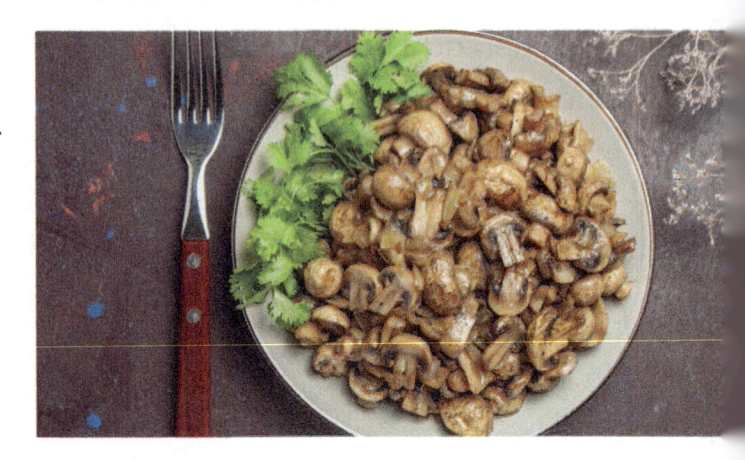

# Almond-Crusted Mahi-Mahi

## Ingredients

- 1 tablespoon ground almonds
- 2 tablespoons grated parmesan cheese
- 1 tablespoon breadcrumbs
- 5 ounces mahi-mahi
- 3 tablespoons plain Greek yogurt, divided
- Juice of 1 lemon
- 1 teaspoons fresh or ½ teaspoon of dried dill, divided, plus extra as garnish (optional)
- Salt and pepper

## Preparation Method

1. Preheat oven to 400°F. Line a baking sheet with parchment paper and set it aside.

2. In a small bowl, toss together the almonds, parmesan, breadcrumbs, and half the dill to combine. Season with a little black pepper.

3. Season each piece of the mahi-mahi with salt and pepper. Place on baking sheet.

4. Use a small brush or knife to apply a thin layer of yogurt (1 tablespoon) over the fish. Apply the almond mixture to the tops of the fish using your hands. Gently press down to ensure the coating sticks.

5. Bake for 15-20 minutes until the fish flakes easily.

6. To make the sauce, in a small bowl, combine 2 tablespoons of Greek yogurt with the lemon juice and the rest of the dill. Season with salt and mix well. Refrigerate until ready to use.

7. When the fish is ready, serve with the lemon dill sauce.

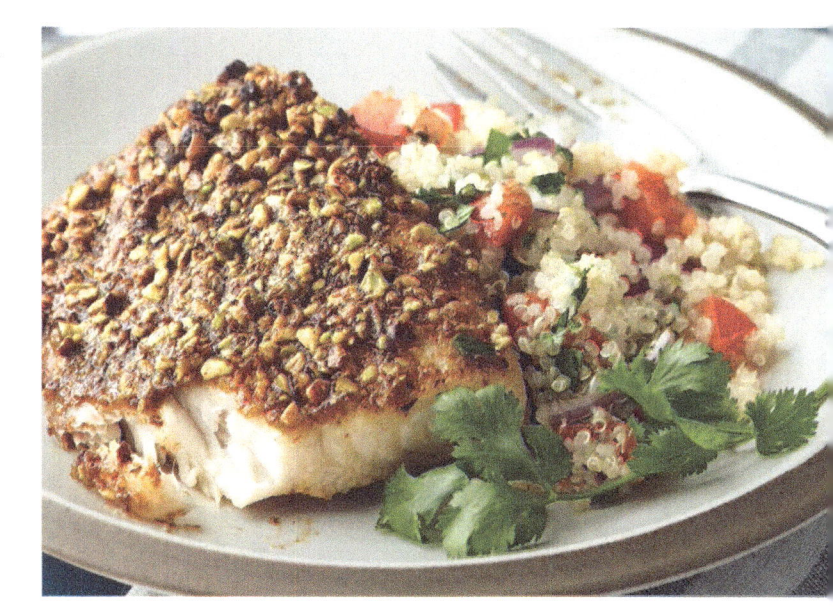

Copyright © 2024 by Dr. Su-Nui Escobar, RDN, LDN

## YOU GOT THIS!

Ready to supercharge your weight loss journey? Join my email list for more meal ideas, expert insights, and the latest research on weight loss medications.

Stay in the loop and get inspired on your path to a healthier you.

Sign up now for exclusive content delivered to your inbox.

Join Our Community

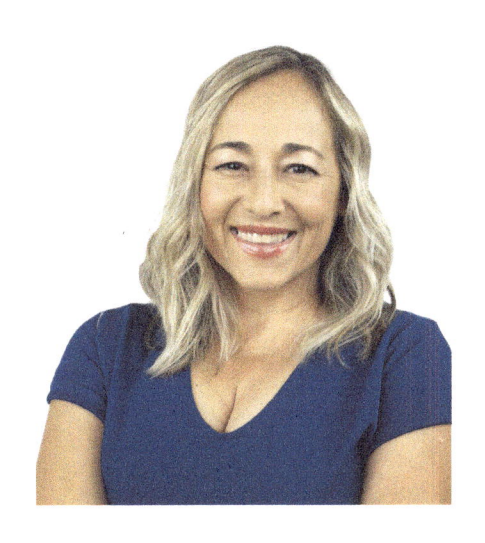

## About Dr. Su-Nui Escobar, DCN, RDN, FAND

My name is Dr. Su-Nui Escobar, and I am a doctor in clinical nutrition and a registered dietitian/nutritionist.

I love helping on their journey through weightloss. In a world saturated with social media trends and fads, I provide practical tips, recipes, ideas to lose weight, improve health based on scientific research.

Follow me at:

nutritionforweightlossmeds.com

Made in the USA
Las Vegas, NV
14 September 2024